The Premed Playbook

Guide to the Medical School Application Process

ENDORSEMENTS

"I love this book! It is complete in its coverage of topics related to the medical school application and admission process. I can easily see prospective applicants picking it up and getting a great overview of what is involved. It is an excellent resource for applicants as they make their way through the gruesome admissions journey. I can also imagine students giving a copy of the book to friends and family members who don't know anything about the process to introduce them to what students will be facing in the weeks and months of their application cycle. It is straightforward in addressing the more nuanced and difficult topics sometimes faced by students. Dr. Gray has established a reputation for being honest and frank with students, and I believe this book continues that legacy."

—**James Scott Wright, EdD**, Vice President for Academic Advising, Mappd, LLC, Retired Executive Director, Texas Medical and Dental Schools Application Service, Former Director of Admissions, UT Southwestern Medical School

"The instruction manual that the premedical community has needed is finally here! This book is a comprehensive resource for all aspects of the application to medical school. In addition to the clear advice that Dr. Gray provides, he offers examples of strong and weak responses and, most importantly, why they are strong or weak."

—**Leila Amiri, PhD**, Assistant Dean for Admissions & Recruitment, University of Illinois Chicago College of Medicine Co-Chair AAMC BA/MD Affiliate Group

"This Guide to the Medical School Application Process is a very practical tool for medical school applicants, especially for those new to this journey. Dr. Gray included the hottest topics in the premed world, so reading this book would equip most with everything they need to navigate this journey successfully. Although this book is designed for applicants, the content is very relevant to all premed students. If there were a Premed 101 college course, this would be the textbook!"

—**Joanne Snapp, MSEd**, Former Director of Health Professions Advising, University of California, Davis, Former Director of Admissions, Donald and Barbara Zucker School of Medicine at Hofstra/Northwell

"What a wonderfully thorough and comprehensive resource! Dr. Gray has provided a very thoughtful and methodical approach to the medical school application. Through a multitude of examples, he demonstrates how to highlight one's passions and strengths while avoiding common pitfalls that are easy to make. *The Premed Playbook Guide to the Medical School Application Process* is much more than a compilation of dos and don'ts. It's a fun and easy read that will help applicants navigate each part of the process and stay on track during a very busy and sometimes stressful time in their professional journey!"

—**Gregory M. Polites, MD, FACEP,** Associate Professor of Emergency Medicine, Chair, Central Subcommittee on Admissions, Washington University School of Medicine

"The challenge today is there's just too much information available on the topic of admission to medical school. However, Dr. Gray synthesizes the most essential concepts and principles into his latest book with authentic examples to help demystify the entire process."

—**Joon Kim, EdD**, Senior Program Director of Postbaccalaureate Programs, Keck Graduate Institute

THE PREMED PLAYBOOK

GUIDE TO THE MEDICAL SCHOOL APPLICATION PROCESS

Everything You Need to Successfully Apply

RYAN GRAY, MD

NEW YORK

LONDON • NASHVILLE • MELBOURNE • VANCOUVER

The Premed Playbook Guide to the Medical School Application Process

Everything You Need to Successfully Apply

Published in New York, New York, by Morgan James Publishing. Morgan James is a trademark of Morgan James, LLC. www.MorganJamesPublishing.com

ISBN 9781631955235 paperback
ISBN 9781631955242 ebook
Library of Congress Control Number:
2021931722

Cover Design by:
DesignerName
www.website.com

Interior Design by:
DesignerName
www.website.com

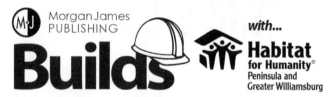

Morgan James is a proud partner of Habitat for Humanity Peninsula and Greater Williamsburg. Partners in building since 2006.

Get involved today! Visit
MorganJamesPublishing.com/giving-back

To my son, Ethan. You have added more love and light to our family than I could have ever imagined

TABLE OF CONTENTS

ACKNOWLEDGMENTS

As with my previous books, this book would not have been possible without the hundreds of students who submitted their essays and sacrificed their time to do mock interviews with me. Without their efforts, this book would not have been as helpful to you on your journey. This is the epitome of *Collaboration, Not Competition*. If you want to be part of an amazing community of premeds, go to premedhangout.com.

INTRODUCTION

How many times have you thought about opening up that email or receiving that phone call congratulating you on getting into medical school? Every year, more than 60,000 premed students apply for a seat in medical school. For some, the process ends with tears of joy and excitement. For others, it brings tears of sadness, as they don't receive any acceptances.

Why did the accepted students get in, and what could the rejected students have done to improve their chances? In this book, *The Premed Playbook: Guide to the Medical School Application*, we'll cover everything you need to know to help you put together a strong application. First impressions are important, and your primary application is the first impression you're going to make to the Admissions Committees.

I've experienced both situations. The first year I applied to medical school, I didn't get in. I thought my career as a physician was over even before it started. The reality was that my application was not strong enough yet. This is the same reality for half, if not more, of all applicants to med school—the need to reapply.

Unfortunately, many students are applying without knowing how to put forward the best application. That is why I wrote this book.

The Premed Playbook: Guide to the Medical School Application isn't going to change your GPA. It can't change your MCAT score. This book can't improve your extracurriculars or give you research that you've never done. It also is not here to replace the instruction manuals for each of the application services; those are invaluable in answering your specific and unique questions about each part of the application. My hope is that this book will draw attention to areas of the application that need even more attention.

What you can expect from this book is a resource to turn to as you are completing your medical school applications. It will be here when you have questions about how to write your extracurricular descriptions or which extracurriculars to include when you are out of space. It will be here when you're trying to narrow down your school list and to help you understand the budgeting around applying to medical school. This book will take you from thinking about the application to having all the information you need to help you put together your best application and, hopefully, secure a spot in a medical school where you will thrive.

Many students underestimate the importance of a strong application and only focus on their GPA and MCAT score. I don't want you to make that mistake, and if you are reading this, you won't.

I don't expect you to sit down and read this book all the way through from start to finish. I encourage you to keep it near you as you are working on each part of your application. However, I do want you to read one chapter right now—the next one. After that, you will have some insight into how to best apply to medical school, and from there, you can go to each relevant chapter for the current part of the application you are working on.

My goal is to prevent you from needing to reapply to medical school based on common, avoidable mistakes. I want you to be as prepared as possible when it comes to submitting your application. I want you to feel confident when you click the "submit" button and spend the thousands of dollars that it can cost to apply to schools, travel for interviews, and pay all of the extra costs that come with the process.

Applying to medical school is expensive. If I can prevent you from needing to reapply to medical school, then I know the small investment in this book will be worthwhile. Let's go ahead and get started by jumping into some of the biggest takeaways that I need you to know right now before you even start thinking about the medical school application.

QUICK TAKEAWAYS

When 50% of students don't have a successful application cycle, the common question is "why?" What prevented those students from getting an acceptance, or maybe even an interview?

When speaking to students and hearing stories of their struggles, they are often making very common mistakes that stand in the way of their success in the application cycle. With so much information out there, it breaks my heart to see students who I know would make competent and caring physicians quickly overlooked due to a "fatal" mistake in their application. If they had the proper knowledge, there's no doubt in my mind they would have had a much better chance of getting into medical school.

In this chapter, I will lay out the most common areas where students make mistakes, or have misconceptions, that can negatively affect their application. My hope is that, even if this is the only chapter you read, you're going to be a more successful applicant because of it. As you read the rest of the book, we will dive even further into each of these areas and I will help you craft your application to create an outstanding first impression.

Timing of the Application

Not applying early is the number one preventable mistake students make every year. I partly blame the medical schools and the application services for this continued mistake. Students, up to this point in their academic career, live off of deadlines. They have deadlines for their assignments in class. They have deadlines when it comes to applying to undergrad institutions. They have deadlines for everything in this world, and so when it comes to applying to medical school, they look at those deadlines and they say, "Okay, my deadline is October 31st. As long as I have everything done by then, my MCAT by then, I am good." This is false. Deadlines for the medical school application process need to be, have to be, 100% ignored.

The application cycle, for most med schools, is based on a rolling admissions process, which means Admissions Committees review applications and extend interview invites as they come in. Therefore, the longer you wait to submit your application, the harder it can be for you to receive an interview invite, and the harder it will be for you to ultimately receive an acceptance.

To increase your chances of success, you need to apply as early as possible in the application cycle. I consider a late application to be any application not fully complete (including, but not limited to, MCAT scores, secondaries, and letters of recommendation) by the end of August. An entire chapter on the application timeline will be explored later in the book.

Application Services

There are three application services in the United States: AMCAS, AACOMAS, and TMDSAS. You can apply to one, two, or all three of the application services at the same time, as they all serve different medical schools, including allopathic (MD) medical schools (AMCAS), osteopathic (DO) medical schools (AACOMAS), and Texas public medical schools (both MD and DO schools) (TMDSAS). Starting in 2021, TMDSAS also includes Baylor College of Medicine, the only private medical school included. Each of them has its own nuances, which will be covered in the different sections of this book.

The Personal Statement

The personal statement is one of the biggest headaches for most premed students. This is not an essay about the skills or traits that are going to make you a great physician. This is not an essay about the bad experience you had as a patient and why you want to be better than those physicians. This is not an essay in which you write out your résumé in paragraph format. This is an essay about *why* you want to be a doctor.

One of the biggest mistakes you can make when it comes to writing the personal statement is waiting until the last minute because you think it is going to be easy to write about yourself and you'll throw something together. This affects your ability to get an interview invite to medical school.

In a later chapter, I will discuss the personal statement in-depth and provide many examples to help guide you in writing yours. Additionally, I have a whole book dedicated to the personal statement in this Premed Playbook series, *The Premed Playbook: Guide to the Medical School Personal Statement.*

The MCAT

The Medical College Admission Test®, or MCAT®, is an almost eight-hour-long beast of a test. Almost every medical school requires it to be considered for admission. Because of rolling admissions, you want your MCAT score to be in as soon as possible. The latest I would recommend taking the MCAT is March or April of the year in which you are applying to medical school. It takes about a month to get your score, so if you take it around that time, you should have your score back before you submit your application. The timing helps if you need to retake the exam as well, letting you schedule a new test date without hurting your application timing too much. If you are thinking about taking the MCAT after July, I would discuss this with your advisor to see if you should delay your application.

We will have a lot more on the MCAT later on in this book, and I also have a full book dedicated to it, *The Premed Playbook: Guide to the MCAT.*

GPA

Your GPA is a big part of the application, and it gives medical schools confidence that you will be able to handle their curriculum. The GPA your school calculates is oftentimes different than the GPA the application service calculates. Also, when filling out your application, every single class you've taken, even if replaced on your college transcript, must be included and calculated as part of your GPA. You can go to whatsmygpa.com to see what your med school application GPA will be.

Your GPA is broken down into science and non-science classes as well as undergraduate (which includes dual-enrollment high school courses and undergraduate classes taken after your bachelor's degree, i.e., postbac) and graduate classes.

Minimum GPAs and MCAT scores

Medical schools receive thousands of applications per application cycle, necessitating an easy way to make sure they are inviting the best applicants for their school. Passing the boards the first time and finishing medical school in four years are key metrics that medical schools are evaluated on by the accreditation bodies. One of the quickest ways to determine if you are academically capable of doing this is to make sure you meet their set minimum academic requirements.

Unfortunately, most medical schools are not transparent with their cutoffs and don't publish these numbers. The customary minimum stats to apply are a 3.0 GPA and a 500 MCAT. Even with that said, if you listen to my podcast, *The Premed Years*, you'll hear many stories of students who did not meet those minimums who were still accepted into medical school. I will talk about GPA and MCAT much more later on.

Letters of Recommendation

When applying to medical school, you will need to ask former professors, physicians who know you well, and others for a letter of recommendation (or evaluation). Your application will usually not be considered complete unless these letters have been submitted. I've heard horror stories from students who had to wait for months for a letter of recommendation to be submitted, causing them to lose out on an interview invite.

Therefore, you should start requesting letters of recommendation early in the application cycle to give your letter writers time to compose a strong letter. If you are using a third-party service, like Interfolio, to store your letters, you can start asking for them before the application cycle opens. If you are using the application service, as of right now, your letter writers can't submit a letter until the new application cycle opens.

As for the amount and type of letters you need, a general rule of thumb is to have at least three: two from science professors and one from a non-science professor. However, every medical school has its own requirements, so you should look at the schools you are applying to and make sure you have what they want.

The Committee Letter

If your undergrad institution has a committee letter, you should open up a dialogue with the committee about a year before you are planning on applying to find out what they require to receive a letter. Your advising office needs to know who you are (you'd be surprised how many students don't seek out any help until the application cycle starts), and you need to know who they are as well as the resources they have to support you. You also need to understand the requirements they may have to work with students. For example, some advising offices will not work with students or write committee letters unless the student meets certain GPA and MCAT cutoffs set by the advising office.

If you do not qualify for a committee letter, or you are not at a school that offers one, you will apply to medical school with individual letters from your letter writers.

Activities

As you progress through your premed career, everything you do might end up in the activities section of the application. As with most other parts of the application, each application service has different requirements for your activities. Applying to medical school with amazing stats sometimes will not overcome a lack of specific activities, namely shadowing and clinical experience.

Many students look at their activities as a series of checkboxes. Make sure you show consistency in your experiences, so it doesn't look like you are only trying to meet the minimums you think are necessary to show med schools you want to be a doctor.

Secondary Applications

After your primary application is submitted, most schools will send you what is known as a secondary application. This application is generally one to four (or more) essay topics. You'll need to budget both time and money for these secondaries.

Since it is important to submit your secondary applications as soon as possible (generally within two weeks), an important strategy to handle the burden of writing the secondary application essays is to pre-write them. Most schools do not change their essay topics from year to year. You can see our secondary essay database at secondaryapps.com.

School List

There are a few different types of medical schools in the US—public and private. Since public schools are state funded, there is usually a mandate in place as to the number of out-of-state students the med school can accept. Texas public schools can only accept a maximum of 10% of their students from out of state. The University of Michigan is one of the few exceptions to public schools and the numbers of in-state versus out-of-state enrollment. The Medical School Admissions Requirements (MSAR) platform offered by the Association of American Medical Colleges (AAMC) shows the numerical breakdown of students interviewed and accepted from out of state.

Budget

Applying to medical school is expensive. Make sure you are ready for the financial burden of the applications by saving as much money as possible. You should also look into the Fee Assistance Programs offered by the AAMC and American Association of Colleges of Osteopathic Medicine (AACOM) to help offset some of the costs of the application and the MCAT. You can go to appexpenses.com to get an estimate of the cost of applying to medical school.

Conclusion

These are some of the common topics that I see students failing to understand prior to getting involved in the medical school application process. I hope I've given you the start to a solid foundation so you know what you should be doing to help you prepare for your medical school application.

DEFINITIONS

There is a lot of jargon that gets thrown around the premed world and beyond. The last thing I want is for you to miss a crucial aspect of the medical school application process because you don't understand one of these definitions. Let's tackle some of them here. This is just an introduction to the language you may see here and elsewhere throughout the application cycle. We'll cover most of these in further detail in the rest of the book.

Primary Application

The medical school application is typically broken down into a primary application and a secondary application. When students think about applying to medical school, they are likely thinking only about the primary application, which is really three different applications depending on where you are applying. The Texas Medical and Dental School Application Service (TMDSAS) is the country's oldest application service and serves the public medical schools (MD and DO, vet, dental, and more) in the state of Texas. It now (starting in 2021) also supports Baylor College of Medicine, which is a private medical school in

Texas. The American Medical Colleges Application Service® (AMCAS®) is the largest application service and serves the allopathic (MD) medical schools, except for public Texas MD schools. The Association of American Colleges of Osteopathic Medicine Application Service (AACOMAS®) is the youngest of the application services and is used to apply to osteopathic (DO) medical schools, except for public Texas DO schools. Some students apply to just one of the three application services. Some apply to two of the three, and others will apply to all three services.

Secondary Application

After you submit your primary application, most schools will send you a secondary application, typically through email or through the school's specific website or application portal. Some schools screen applicants before sending a secondary application. Screening is usually done to determine if a student is academically qualified for that specific school. Most secondary applications require you to write and submit additional essays, as well as pay a fee. If you qualify for the Fee Assistance Program (FAP), most schools will waive the secondary fee. Secondaryapps.com is updated each year with the new prompts schools send out as soon as we get them from students.

Fee Assistance Programs

Both the AAMC and AACOM® offer Fee Assistance Programs (FAP). Please review their qualification guidelines and application timelines, and make sure you apply early if you are eligible. To apply for the financial assistance program, you need to have access to your tax returns as well as your parents' returns, regardless of your age or dependency status.

AAMC

The Fee Assistance Program through the AAMC will help with the cost of taking the MCAT, as well as the cost of applying to medical schools. It significantly reduces the registration costs of the MCAT and offers the AAMC MCAT prep materials for free. FAP also reduces the cost of the AMCAS application and allows the applicant to apply to the first 20 schools for free. If you want to apply to more than 20 schools, you need to pay the fee for each additional school. Your FAP status is sent to the medical schools where you've applied through AMCAS, and most, if not all, will waive your secondary application fees.

AACOM

The Fee Assistance Program through AACOM waives the AACOMAS application fee, which includes the cost of applying to one osteopathic medical school. If you want to apply to more than one school, you need to pay the fee for each additional school.

Gap Year

A gap year is a year (sometimes more than one) that is taken after undergraduate work is complete instead of going directly to medical school. It may be taken when a student postpones their application in order to improve MCAT, GPA, or other developmental parts of their application. Students may also take a gap year if they are not accepted to medical school during their senior year of college. If you start as an undergraduate in August of 2020 and finish in May of 2024, and you apply and are accepted to medical school in a traditional timeline, you will apply for medical school in 2023 and start med school in August of 2024.

If, for some reason, you decide to take a gap year because you want to travel or dedicate more time to studying for the MCAT, or any other reason, you would then apply the year before you want to start medical school. That year (or years) between graduating from undergrad and starting in medical school is known as your gap year(s). Some like to refer to it as a growth year to avoid any negative connotation around the term gap year. You can use your gap year to strengthen your application, to work, to explore, or to rest if you are burned out from your undergrad workload.

Glide Year

Glide year is the term typically used instead of a gap year when referring to students in a postbac. Because of the application timelines and school schedules of the postbac, there is usually an extra year before starting medical school. This is also known as an "application year."

Postbac

Postbaccalaureate, or postbac (or postbac, post-bach, or the many other ways that people spell it), is any sort of coursework that is taken after you finish your undergraduate, or baccalaureate, degree. This is for students who need to either improve their academic record or take the science prerequisites for the first time. Many students whom I talk to don't even know this is an option.

There are formal postbac programs—usually with some form of pre-health advising—that you can apply to, similar to a graduate program. Many formal postbac programs have linkage agreements with medical schools—if you maintain a certain GPA and/or MCAT score in the postbac program, you can be guaranteed an interview, or even an acceptance, at a medical school.

There are also do-it-yourself, or DIY, postbac programs in which you can enroll in courses at any undergraduate institution (four-year or community college) to take extra classes.

Special Master's Program

Similar to a postbac, a Special Master's Program (SMP) is a type of master's program specifically designed for premed or other pre-health professional students. A lot of SMPs are affiliated with medical schools, and classes are taken with first-year medical students. SMPs can be of great assistance when undergrad or postbac records are poor. An SMP may be your last line of defense if you need to prove to the medical schools that you have fixed your study habits.

Rolling Admissions

Rolling admissions is something that gets a lot of students in trouble. Every medical school and application service has deadlines posted; many students assume if they get their application in by the deadline, they have just as much of an opportunity of acceptance as someone who submitted their application when the applications opened. This could not be further from the truth with rolling admissions.

With rolling admissions, used by most schools in the US, the earlier you submit your application, the earlier it is reviewed and a decision is made. If you interview for a seat at a school in August, there are more seats available to you than someone who interviews in December.

It's like a giant game of musical chairs, except with musical chairs, there is always one more player than seats. With rolling admissions, the number of seats decreases with every new acceptance, but the number of players (applicants) increases every day as more students submit their applications.

The moral of the story is you should try to get your applications in as soon as you can.

Prerequisites (Prereqs)

Most medical schools have a set of required courses you must take and pass (usually a "C" grade or better) prior to matriculation, known as prerequisites. You can usually apply to schools and be accepted without meeting the requirements, but you will need them before you start med school. Check with each school for their prerequisites.

GPA

Most students understand what a grade point average, or GPA, is; however, what you might not know is that the GPA you see on your transcripts will probably not be the GPA that is given to the medical schools. Each application service has different requirements for what classes you must report, and each calculates your GPA slightly differently.

Cumulative GPA

Your cumulative GPA, or cGPA, is your total GPA with all of your undergraduate courses included. An overall GPA includes graduate coursework.

Science GPA

Your science GPA, or sGPA, also known as your BCPM (Biology, Chemistry, Physics, Math) GPA for AMCAS and TMDSAS, and your BCP (Biology,

Chemistry, Physics) GPA for AACOMAS, includes the courses that are classified as science courses by each application service.

MSAR

The Medical School Admission Requirements™ (MSAR®) is an online database developed by the AAMC and available through a paid subscription. Students can search, sort, and compare information about US and Canadian medical schools, postbac programs, SMPs, BS/MD programs, and more. In addition to information about the average GPAs and MCAT scores, the MSAR also indicates each school's preferences for prerequisites taken online, at a community college, or obtained through AP credit.

CASPer

CASPer® is a form of situational judgment test. It's an online test taken during the application process to medical school. These tests present the student with hypothetical situations and ask what the student would do in such situations. CASPer requires you to write your answers; it is not a multiple-choice test. Not every school requires the CASPer, and each school's use of the CASPer in their admissions process varies.

CASPer Snapshot

The Altus Assessments team has introduced the CASPer Snapshot, which is a three-question one-way interview tool. This tool is meant to help medical schools understand more about who you are, especially with the limited travel caused by the COVID-19 pandemic.

AAMC SJT

Similar to CASPer, the AAMC SJT is a situational judgment test. Unlike CASPer, the AAMC SJT is multiple choice. It was introduced during the 2020-2021 application cycle at a few test schools.

VITA

The AAMC VITA™, or Virtual Interview Tool for Admissions, is an online platform that asks students to record themselves answering questions. Medical schools utilize it in assessing a student's pre-professional competencies. It was introduced during the 2020-2021 application cycle, though it was previously used and dropped for Emergency Medicine residency applications because it wasn't useful.

Holistic Review

Holistic review is an admissions process used by medical schools to make sure the whole student is being considered. Academic performance, experiences, and personal attributes are all weighed together to determine an applicant's fit for the medical school. While holistic review is not just a buzzword but something most medical schools use, stats are still very important in the admissions process because the first goal of the medical school is to accept students who are capable of getting through the rigorous medical school curriculum and board exams.

Extracurriculars

Extracurriculars, also called your activities, are the things you are doing outside, or sometimes inside, of school. These are the activities that make up what you do with your time, and they don't have to be exclusively healthcare-related. There is a specific section on the application where you will list these.

Clinical Experiences

Clinical experiences are experiences, paid or volunteer, in which you are directly interacting with patients. These include working as an emergency medical technician (EMT), scribe, phlebotomist, or medical assistant, to name a few. Working the front desk at an outpatient clinic or in registration for the Emergency Department are not clinical experiences. Working as a janitor in a hospital is not considered clinical experience. Yes—I had a student put this in their application because they thought being in the hospital automatically meant it was a clinical experience.

Shadowing

Shadowing is a separate category in the activity section of the application. Shadowing is not clinical experience, and vice versa. Shadowing is following a physician around to see what their day looks like.

Volunteering

Volunteering, for the purposes of the application, is usually talked about in non-clinical terms. Things like Habitat for Humanity, volunteering at the local shelter, etc., are what we are referring to when we talk about volunteering. Remember that clinical experience can be a volunteer or paid position.

Multiple Mini Interview (MMI)

The MMI is an interview format originally created at McMaster University in Canada by the same people who created the CASPer. It was first used in 2004. It is a station-based interview format in which the interviewee is given a situational question and asked to enter the station and respond. The MMI is supposed to remove a lot of bias from the interview process.

Admissions Committee

The Admissions Committee, or adcom, is the group of people who decide who gets into each medical school class. There are usually many more people who help with interviewing who are not on the Admissions Committee.

Letter of Recommendation or Letter of Evaluation

A letter of recommendation (LOR) is a document that you request from several different people throughout the application cycle. Each school has different requirements in terms of what LORs they want.

Early Decision (EDP)

Early Decision is a special application pathway for students who want to apply to only one school; the hope is that the one school will interview and accept you. Not every medical school participates in EDP.

Underrepresented in Medicine

Underrepresented in Medicine (URM) is a term created by *Project 3000 by 2000 -- Racial and Ethnic Diversity in U.S. Medical Schools* and defined by the AAMC as "those racial and ethnic populations that are underrepresented in the medical profession relative to their numbers in the general population." This describes how Admissions Committees view one's ethnicity or race[1]. Currently, there is no set definition for URM, as every medical school can interpret it how they want based on their own population demographics.

Overrepresented in Medicine

Overrepresented in Medicine (ORM) is a term created by the premed world as the opposite of URM. This terminology is problematic because it tends to imply that being from a dominant, widely represented group makes getting into medical school harder. ORM is not a real thing, and it comes across that you're complaining that you're White, Asian, wealthy, etc.

Allopathic Medicine

Allopathic medicine refers to science-based, modern medicine. MD degree holders are referred to as allopathic physicians.

Osteopathic Medicine

Osteopathic medicine, while still science-based, modern medicine, differs in the degree that the physician holds. These physicians hold DO degrees.

Osteopathic Manipulative Medicine (OMM)/Osteopathic Manipulative Treatment (OMT)

According to the Association of American Colleges of Osteopathic Medicine, OMT can be used to treat structural and functional issues in the bones, joints, tissues, and muscles of the body. It uses the relationship between the neuromusculoskeletal system and the rest of the body to restore functionality

---

1   https://www.aamc.org/what-we-do/diversity-inclusion/underrepresented-in-medicine

and/or remove barriers to motion and healing while achieving and maintaining the patient's health as part of a whole system of evaluation and treatment.

Matriculant

A student who has entered into a school and started is a matriculant. This is in contrast to an accepted student. A student could be accepted to five schools, but they will only matriculate into one.

International Medical Graduate (IMG)

Formerly known as Foreign Medical Graduates (FMGs), IMGs are students who go to medical school outside of the US or Puerto Rico.

Pre-match and Match for TMDSAS

The TMDSAS application process includes what is known as the pre-match and match. The pre-match is very similar to every other school or application service, with schools offering acceptances to students. The match is very similar to *The Match* for residency programs—TMDSAS's match program has students rank their top choice schools where they interviewed. Then the schools rank the students, and a computer algorithm pairs the students with schools based on each other's rankings. The pre-match and match process is only for Texas residents. Non-Texas residents are accepted throughout a standard rolling admissions process.

Red Flags

A red flag is a generic term for anything that may cause any issues on your application. Things like arrests, institutional actions, big gaps in your education, or very poor grades could be considered red flags.

Dual-Degree Programs

Many, if not most, medical schools offer some sort of dual-degree program at their institution. Programs like MD(DO)/PhD, MD(DO)/MBA, and MD(DO)/MPH are all examples of dual-degree programs.

Nontraditional Applicant

A nontraditional applicant (nontrad) is someone who did not go straight from high school to college to medical school. A nontrad could be someone changing careers or someone who decided to take some time before applying to medical school.

Verification Process

After submitting an application, each of the application services will verify the information—most notably the course and grade information. For AMCAS and AACOMAS, this process takes time and is done before schools have access to your data. TMDSAS verifies after the data is sent to schools.

Disadvantaged Student

The AMCAS application asks if you want to consider yourself a disadvantaged student. The definition of a disadvantaged student is appropriately very vague to give each student the opportunity to discuss their story.

APPLICATION TIMELINE

Now that you know about all of the medical school application services, let's talk about the timing of everything. This is probably one of the most important chapters in the whole book. It is not a sexy chapter about how to write a killer personal statement or how to crush your extracurriculars. It is not about the secrets of applying to different schools. This chapter is going to lay out the timeline of every step of the overall application process. In subsequent chapters, we will dive further into timelines for each part of the application, like transcripts, letters of recommendation, and personal statements.

When Does the Application Open?

Every year, the cycle of premed life continues with the closing of one cycle and the opening of another. In fact, the application cycle is so long that some medical schools are still sending out their final acceptances even as new applicants are starting to fill out and submit applications for the next class.

Hopefully you remember from the Quick Takeaways chapter that you should get your application in as soon as possible because the application cycle for most schools is based on rolling admissions. The later you apply, the lower your chances of getting an acceptance.

Application services open at the beginning of May for each class that will start in July or August of the following year. For example, if you are planning on starting medical school in August 2030, you would want to start filling out your application in May of 2029. The length of the application cycle is something that throws a lot of students off and causes them to rush to complete an application they did not think they had to do until the following year.

AMCAS has historically had a delay between when the application opens and when you can actually submit your application. After opening in early May, students take that month to fill out all of the information and essays needed and then submit at the end of May or the beginning of June. I recommend following AMCAS and the AAMC on all of their social media channels to stay up to date with everything they are doing.

AACOMAS also opens in early May, but unlike AMCAS, you can submit your application right away. Slow down, though; every year, students submit their applications without them actually being complete. You have to know that once you submit your application, you cannot change it (with a few exceptions). The submit button is not a "save and come back later" button.

Starting in 2021, TMDSAS will also have a delay between when the application opens and when you can submit the application.

What is the Primary Application Deadline?

Deadlines for the primary applications in AMCAS and AACOMAS are set by each of the participating schools. TMDSAS has set its deadline as the beginning of October. Deadlines are very strict, and you should not delay.

A simple web search of AMCAS deadlines will bring you to AMCAS' page with every medical school's deadline. The dates historically range from mid-October to mid-December, with a few outliers. The most popular deadline for AMCAS schools is November 1st.

AACOMAS deadlines can be found in the Student Guide to Osteopathic Medicine. The most popular deadline for AACOMAS schools is March 1st, the year after applications open.

Please remember that deadlines should never be missed, nor ignored. To be seriously considered for an interview, you need to have your application submitted as soon as possible. Speaking with a Dean of Admissions at one school, she said: "We practically filled the class after the first admissions committee meeting." Again, every school will be different in how and when they fill their class, but the majority of schools are based on rolling admissions and, therefore, the earlier you submit, the better your chances will be.

Can I Submit Without Completing Everything?

There are many parts of the application that do not need to be completed before you submit your application. For example, if you are planning on taking the MCAT in late June, I would still recommend submitting your application as soon as you can. Getting in line for verification (explained below) is important. You don't want to wait until your score comes back in late July to submit. Submitting your application at that stage can delay verification until late August or even September.

You don't need all of your letters of recommendation to be collected before you submit your application, either.

You will need your essays and activities to be completed prior to submitting your application. These sections cannot be edited once submitted.

You will need to select at least one school to submit your application. You can add more schools later.

What Happens After I Submit My Application?

After you submit your application, each application service to which you applied needs to verify your information. This is a manual process of comparing your transcripts to what you entered, which is why the verification process can take up to six weeks in some extreme cases. The later you apply, the farther back in line you are to be verified.

Picture the lines at a sporting event where everyone has brought a huge backpack full of junk, and security has to check each one by hand. If you're getting to the game right before the first pitch, you'll be in line for a while. Show up an hour earlier, and you'll likely walk right up to the checkpoint.

Historically, the AMCAS verification process is the longest, likely because they receive the most applications. When you read about long verification process times, I'm likely referring to the AMCAS process. If you're only applying to DO schools, the verification process is usually much shorter, but you should still apply as early as you can because of rolling admissions.

TMDSAS processes and verifies applications throughout the application cycle after schools see your application, and potentially after your interviews. Just in case you thought you might be able to slip something by the verifiers, every year, students are found falsifying information in the applications; this is then reported to the schools and the other application services.

When Do Schools Receive My Application?

You would think once you submit your application that medical schools would start pounding on your door to have you submit your secondary essays. This isn't the case, especially if you submit early.

Both AMCAS and AACOMAS hold all early applications and send them to medical schools as a batch to kick off the cycle. AMCAS has historically sent out the first wave of applications to medical schools at the end of June. AACOMAS is usually a couple of weeks ahead, sending out their first batch in mid-June. Before this first batch of applications, medical schools cannot see that you have applied to their school and therefore cannot send you a secondary application. TMDSAS is different and doesn't hold the applications back to send in a batch.

If you submitted your application on June 1st, you will likely not hear anything until that first batch goes out. This is the perfect time to start looking at secondary essays!

When Will I Receive Secondary Applications?

If you submitted your application early (the importance of which I can't stress enough), you won't get secondaries back from DO schools until mid-June, and you'll hear nothing from MD schools until late June. This delay is the perfect time to start pre-writing your secondary essays, so you are not overwhelmed when they start coming in. You can find an updated list of secondary essay prompts at secondaryapps.com. If you find a school has updated its prompts, please submit those new prompts to updatesecondaries.com.

If you submit your AMCAS or AACOMAS application after the first batch of applications goes out, medical schools can "see" your application and that you've identified them as a school where you are applying. This means they can send you a secondary application. That doesn't mean they will. Some schools may wait until you are verified before sending you a secondary application.

Will I Get a Secondary Application from Every School?

Yes. No. Maybe. As we go through this process, you'll see me hedge on most questions with an answer of *it depends*. Contingent on the schools you apply to, you might get secondaries back from all of them, or you might not. Some schools screen the primary applications and only send secondary applications to students who are qualified candidates for their school—meaning they meet some minimum standard, usually for GPA and MCAT. Most schools, unfortunately, do not screen and send secondaries to every student who submits a primary application.

Do not assume that because you received a secondary, the school "likes" you, and you have a chance at that school. Just because they didn't screen your application for a secondary doesn't mean your GPA and MCAT are high enough to be reviewed.

You should plan to turn around your secondary applications in two weeks.

CASPer

We will dive into CASPer later on in the book, but I want to briefly mention it in this chapter since many schools use it as part of their secondary application process. Double-check the schools you are applying to and see if they require students to take the CASPer. If they do, register for it as soon as you can. Don't worry; it's not something you have to prepare for—it is just something else to pay for.

When Will I Be Invited for an Interview?

For most schools, your application needs to be complete before they will review it to determine if they want to invite you for an interview. A complete application is one in which you have a verified primary application, completed secondary application (including the CASPer (see later chapter) for schools that require it), all letters of recommendation have been submitted, and all of your MCAT scores have been received. The earlier your application is completed, the earlier schools can review it to determine if they want to invite you for an interview.

Schools receive thousands upon thousands of applications every year and need some way to determine who they want to look at first. One of the easiest things for schools to do is to sort the applications by MCAT and GPA. The stronger your stats, the earlier your application will likely be reviewed. Schools know if your stats and the rest of your application is strong, you'll likely receive a lot of interviews, so they want first dibs. If you're in this bucket, you may start receiving interview invites in July. The majority of schools will start sending out invites in August. Don't plan on any trips during this time!

As the application process goes on, schools start to make their way down the list. If they still have interviews to hand out, and your stats are on the lower side, you should anticipate interviews a little later on in the cycle. It's not unheard of to get an interview as late as March. Many schools at this point in the cycle are interviewing for their waitlist, but an interview is an interview. It's an opportunity to connect with the school and the admissions committee, and you shouldn't pass it up if you don't have any acceptances yet. Even if you're likely not going to get an acceptance this year, a late interview will give you a connection to the school that might make the difference the next time you apply.

When Do Acceptances Come?

Waiting is the hardest part of the application cycle. You wait for it to open. You wait for the secondaries to come. You wait for the interview invites. You wait for the acceptance.

For MD schools, the AAMC asks medical schools not to release their first wave of acceptances until mid-October. This is why if you follow a lot of premed students on social media or in the forums, you'll see students start posting their acceptances at this time. If you're lucky enough to have an August interview at an MD school, the earliest you will hear anything is mid-October, unless you applied Early Decision (more on that later).

For DO applicants, the AOA hasn't asked schools to delay notifying students. Your acceptance might come a week after your interview—or it might come a month after your interview.

Every school will be different as far as when they review their applicants and interviewees and when they accept students. Some schools will wait to interview everybody before they make acceptance decisions, while other schools will make acceptance decisions on a weekly or biweekly basis after every interview cohort. When you are at your interview, the school will typically let you know when to expect to hear something. However, if they don't tell you, you can ask.

The TMDSAS acceptance process is very different from the rest. TMDSAS schools have a match process, similar to what you'll see for residency applications. Out-of-state applicants are not eligible for the match. If you are not a Texas resident, acceptance offers will not begin until October 15th.

TMDSAS Pre-match and Match

TMDSAS has a unique process of accepting Texas residents. Non-residents are not eligible for the match. The pre-match process allows schools to offer a guaranteed acceptance between mid-November and the end of December. This is similar to the other application services. Even if a student pre-matches, they will submit a rank list in the match.

At the beginning of August, students must rank the schools where they have interviewed. Each school will also rank the students who have been interviewed at their school. The rank list is available to students beginning around August 1st, with a deadline to submit the final rankings around mid-January.

If you pre-matched at the second and third schools on your list, but you still want an acceptance to your top choice school, your application will remain open at that top school. You may receive an acceptance during the admissions process that follows the match as students accept and decline offers at different schools. Match results are usually announced at the beginning of February.

AMCAS Choose Your Medical School Tool

New for the 2018-2019 cycle, AMCAS rolled out the "Choose your Medical School Tool." Starting around mid-February, if you're holding an acceptance, you can select "Plan to Enroll" in your AMCAS application. This helps medical schools understand the total number of students who might be part of their class. "Plan to Enroll" allows you to remain on the waitlist for a school that may be higher on your list, or even continue to receive interviews and other acceptances. If you receive an acceptance from a school you'd rather go to, you can change that in your AMCAS application.

The "Plan to Enroll" system does not remove you from schools. You need to let the other schools know you would like to withdraw your application and acceptance from their school if you have been accepted to a school you would rather attend. Doing this will allow schools to offer an acceptance to another student.

At the end of April, you'll have to select either "Plan to Enroll" or "Commit to Enroll." When you select "Commit to Enroll," you are indicating this is your final selection, and you have withdrawn all other AMCAS school applications.

One of the most important things to keep in mind with this new tool is that medical schools are updating their own policies around waitlists and acceptances, and you need to be keenly aware of those as these dates are approaching.

APPLICATION BASICS

Now that we've covered the timeline of the application, let's cover some of the basics.

How Much Does the Medical School Application Cost?

The cost of the entire application process can be a big financial burden for many students. We will have a chapter about the complete cost of the process and tips to budget and pay for the application.

Both AMCAS and AACOMAS charge a base fee for the first school and additional fees for each additional school.

At the time of this writing, AMCAS fees are $170 for the first school and $41 for each additional school. AACOMAS fees are $196 for the first school and $46 for each additional school. TMDSAS charges a flat fee of $185, and you can apply to as many schools as you want.

If you want to know the most up-to-date fees, text APPFEES to 44222 (in the US only), and my system will text you back the current fee structure.

Creating an Account

To submit an application, you'll need to create a single account with each service you plan on using. Go to the following links to create accounts with each service:

AMCAS: medicalschoolhq.net/amcasacct

AACOMAS: medicalschoolhq.net/aacomasacct

TMDSAS: medicalschoolhq.net/tmdsasacct

To submit your application, you'll need a lot of information about your premed path, including some essays and a description of activities you've done as a premed that you want medical schools to know about.

Application Components

The basic information you'll need for each of the applications will be very similar.

Who You Are

You'll need a lot of personal and demographic information including, but not limited to:

- Your legal and preferred names
- Sex and gender identity
- Race and ethnicity
- Birth location and citizenship status
- Family information, including your parent's education levels, jobs, household income, and number of siblings
- Current address and contact information
- Military records
- Convictions
- Language proficiency
- Institutional discipline, for either academic performance or student conduct violations
- License infractions (if you currently or have ever held a professional certification, registration, license, or clinical privileges and had these revoked, suspended, or restricted)

Disadvantaged

For AMCAS, you'll have the opportunity to designate yourself as a disadvantaged applicant. If you say yes, you will have 1325 characters to discuss why you consider yourself disadvantaged. There is a chapter with examples later on in the book.

Nontraditional

If you consider yourself a nontraditional applicant, TMDSAS gives you 500 characters to explain why.

Where You've Been

Each of the application services will want to know your high school and college journey. TMDSAS also asks for your SAT and/or your ACT scores.

Many students have tumultuous college careers, even stopping and starting again at many different institutions. You must be prepared to include every post-secondary (after high school) institution that you've attended, even if the credits transferred, you withdrew, or no credit was earned. This includes courses like EMT training or military training. It also can include study abroad and includes dual-enrollment courses taken while still in high school.

Unfortunately, the transcript portion of the application is a manual process. The technology is not advanced enough yet for every school system to use the same process to supply the data to the application services. AACOMAS has a service to enter your transcript data for you, but I would highly encourage you to do it yourself. I have heard of too many mistakes from this process negatively impacting students.

You'll also need to be prepared to list your major, any minors earned, and the degrees you've earned along the way.

If you have previously matriculated at a medical school, either in the US or abroad, you will also have to explain why you are reapplying to medical school. You'll have 500 characters on the AACOMAS application and 1325 characters on the AMCAS application.

What You've Done

Each of the application services asks for a list of activities that you've completed, commonly referred to as your extracurricular list, or ECs for short. TMDSAS refers to this list as your personal biography. AACOMAS splits them up a little differently and refers to them separately as experiences and achievements. AMCAS refers to them as the work and activities section. Explore the entire chapter dedicated to the activities section later in this book.

Where You Want to Go

Each of the application services needs to know which medical schools you want to apply to. You have the opportunity to select if you are planning on applying Early Decision or to a dual-degree program as well. I'll talk about Early Decision later on in the book.

Essays

As part of all three application services, you'll be required to submit an essay, commonly referred to as the personal statement. This essay provides the school's Admissions Committee with insight into why you want to be a doctor. While I do cover the personal statement in this book, I also have another book dedicated to solely to it, *The Premed Playbook: Guide to the Medical School Personal Statement.*

TMDSAS also has two additional essays, one that is mandatory and one that is optional.

The current mandatory TMDSAS essay is entitled *Personal Characteristics* with the following prompt: "Learning from others is enhanced in educational settings that include individuals from diverse backgrounds and experiences. Please describe your personal characteristics (background, talents, skills, etc.) or experiences that would add to the educational experience of others."

The current optional TMDSAS essay is entitled *Unique Experience* with the following prompt: "Briefly discuss any unique circumstances or life experiences that are relevant to your application which has not previously been presented." Like many of the "optional" parts of the application, I would highly suggest you consider this required.

CORE COMPETENCIES

Every premed student applying to medical school has one question they want to ask—the one question whose answer they think would allow them to put together the perfect application. What is that question?

"What do Admissions Committees want?"

If only it were that easy—figure out what they want and give it to them. Unfortunately, it's not that easy. Too many students take this approach with their applications—the personal statement, extracurriculars, secondaries, and interviews—and it goes very, very badly.

I want you to know about the core competencies the AAMC has created with medical schools. Many Admissions Committees use these core competencies and build upon them as a basic framework for what students they are going to invite for an interview, and ultimately accept. I'm providing this list not as a checklist, but as a reference to help you understand how an Admissions Committee may look at your application.

Admissions Committees will review every aspect of your application (usually after minimum stats are met), and using the AAMC core competencies, usually together with their own guidelines, determine if you demonstrate the qualities they want to see in their medical students to see if they want to invite you for an interview, and ultimately accept you.

The newest structure of the core competencies is broken down into three categories: pre-professional, thinking and reasoning, and science. While these core competencies have been developed to help guide admissions to medical school, you should not use this as an exhaustive list of what you need to get into medical school or be a successful physician.

Remember, there is no checklist to get into med school. These core competencies are meant to provide you with a framework about how your application may be viewed, to help you determine if you are ready to apply to medical school.

Pre-professional Competencies

The pre-professional competencies are all based around you being a good human being, a strong team player, and adaptable. These are all core to being a strong member of the community and a good future physician.

The nine pre-professional competencies are:

- Service Orientation
- Social Skills
- Cultural Competence
- Teamwork
- Oral Communication
- Ethical Responsibility to Self and Others
- Reliability and Dependability
- Resilience and Adaptability
- Capacity for Improvement

You can see from this list that schools want to see a propensity for being in service to others, and while doing so, being able to communicate with those people. They want to see how you dealt with obstacles when you encountered them because, during your medical training, you are going to encounter more than your fair share of challenges.

Thinking and Reasoning Competencies

It's safe to assume that to be a good physician, you need to have the knowledge and ability to think through complicated scenarios. Having the thinking and critical reasoning skills necessary to be a physician is important and hard to measure in an application outside of your grades and MCAT score. Your writing communication can potentially be examined throughout the numerous essays and descriptions that make up your application, and your scientific inquiry can be seen through some of your experiences. Your interview day may also help with some of these competencies.

The four thinking and reasoning competencies are:
- Critical Thinking
- Quantitative Reasoning
- Scientific Inquiry
- Written Communication

Science Competencies

I tell students all the time that they don't have to love science to be a great physician, or to even get into medical school. You just have to be good enough at science, tolerate it, and do well enough to get in and through medical school. I don't think I'm the first to tell you that the knowledge you will learn and use in medicine is all based on the sciences. Communicating with and connecting with patients goes above and beyond science, but without the foundational knowledge, you are likely not going to make a big impact in their lives.

The two science competencies are:
- Living Systems
- Human Behavior

Summary

Every medical school has its own way of evaluating applicants, and these core competencies aren't here to give you a checklist to make sure you prove each and every one of them. Showing up every day and being intentional with your journey as a premed student will likely help you build each of these competencies. For example, only focusing on being a 4.0 student can sacrifice your ability to build teamwork and communication skills. It could also prevent you from having the experiences necessary to prove to yourself that being a physician is what you want.

PAYING FOR THE APPLICATION

I f there was one thing I wish I could change about the application process, it would be the cost. Reading posts on various forums about students not getting accepted to school and not applying again because of the costs breaks my heart. It seems like the majority of the time I see this, it's an underrepresented minority posting these stories. These are the people we need in medicine to benefit the system and our patients in the future.

Since I can't snap my fingers and make it all free, let's talk about how you can prepare for the costs now and set yourself up for success, at least financially speaking, for your application cycle.

Costs Before the Application

Let's first talk about the costs at each stage of the game. The first thing you have to think about is everything that happens before the application. What do you need to do to make sure you can apply to medical school?

First, you have to take the MCAT. The MCAT cost ($320 at the time of this writing for the initial registration cost) is not an insignificant amount of money.

If you have to cancel or reschedule, be prepared to pay more. To prepare for the MCAT, at a minimum, I would recommend getting access to the AAMC MCAT prep materials ($320 at the time of this writing for the online-only materials). That's another good chunk of change. Many of you are likely going to need to take more practice tests than the scored tests the AAMC provides with their prep materials, and that's going to cost a little bit more money as well. I recommend Blueprint (formerly Next Step Test Prep) full-length practice exams because many students say they are the next best option after the AAMC's exams.

After you factor in the cost of a good set of books, you're looking at almost a thousand dollars to self-study for the MCAT. If you think you may need or want a tutor, or you are looking to take an MCAT course, those costs add up even more.

Of course, there are students who get by spending much less, and hopefully, you can do that as well, but I want to make sure you're prepared for something that most students will use. This is even before we start thinking about applying to medical school. There will be some cost-saving tips in the MCAT chapter.

Cost of the Primary Application

After you've spent money preparing for, taking, and hopefully crushing the MCAT, now is the time for your wallet to become a little lighter. The biggest costs will be a little later, but the cost of the primary application(s) is something you need to be prepared to cover, or else you can't apply to medical school in the first place.

One of the first costs of the primary application will come from requesting transcripts from your school(s). You will almost certainly need to request transcripts from **every** post-secondary (after high school) school that you've attended, even if it was for one class that you did not finish. Please check the instruction manuals for each application service to make sure your application won't be delayed because you aren't reporting your classes and schools correctly.

Letters of recommendation can usually be submitted directly to the application service once they open for the cycle, or you may want to use a service like Interfolio. Be prepared to pay an annual fee or a fee to transmit the letters to the application services once you're ready.

If you are planning on using a professional editing service for any part of your application, that comes at a price, too. These services vary wildly based on the company and their qualifications. You don't have to use these services to put together an amazing application. This book, *The Premed Playbook: Guide to the Medical School Application*, and the other books in my Premed Playbook series, can help you craft your story. For complete transparency, I do have a team of advisors and offer editing services through Mappd at premedfeedback.com.

Each application service has its own associated fees. For TMDSAS, it is a one-time, flat fee to apply to one, or all, of the public Texas medical schools. AMCAS and AACOMAS charge one larger fee for the first school, and then a smaller fee for each additional school.

For the most up-to-date fees, text APPFEES to 44222 (in the US only), and my service will text you back the current fee structure.

Cost of Secondary Applications

After you click submit on your primary application, you might think your credit card can go back in your wallet. Unfortunately, it needs to stay out for a while longer.

Once you submit your primary applications, medical schools will then send you secondary applications. The majority of medical schools will send you a secondary application even if you are not statistically qualified to be a student at that school. Even some of the most prestigious Ivy League schools will send you a secondary application if you have a 2.4 GPA and a 490 MCAT score.

When you submit the secondary application to each school, there's typically a fee associated with that as well. Unlike the primary application, which gets paid directly to the application service, the secondary application fee is paid directly to the school. These fees add up very quickly. Don't get caught not having enough money in the bank or enough credit on your card to submit the application in a timely manner. Secondary application fees range anywhere between $40 and $130, or more. If you qualify for FAP, medical schools will typically waive your secondary fee. We have school-specific information about the essay prompts, fees, and other info at secondaryapps.com.

The CASPer test is a newer part of the application process, which costs money as well. I would consider it part of the secondary application process since most schools use it in that way. There is a fee for the test and a fee to transmit that test to each of the schools you designate. Currently, for CASPer, it is $10 to take the test and $10 to transmit to each school.

Cost of Interviews

After a small lull in money going out, hopefully, you are in a situation in which you will start receiving interview invites. Even though it's unlikely for a student to receive a lot of interviews, the cost of each interview makes this one of the most expensive parts of the application process (assuming you have to travel out of town to go to an interview).

For your medical school interview, you'll need to have a suit. Borrow one if you can't afford one and don't have one already. If traveling out of town, you'll need to purchase plane tickets, a room to stay in (hotel or room share), and you'll need money for local transportation and food. If you are lucky, you might have a friend who is near the school where you're interviewing, and you can crash on their couch. Additionally, some schools have programs that let you stay on a current medical student's couch.

Cost of an Acceptance

At this stage of the application cycle, if you have an acceptance, you should be ecstatic. For some students, though, an acceptance brings terror because along with it typically comes a deposit to hold your spot. Can you imagine getting that phone call and being on top of the world, and then reading the follow-up email that has the deposit amount and deadline to submit it only to realize you don't have that money available?

Osteopathic schools need some work in this area. Many schools have very large, non-refundable deposits with very short deadlines to hold your seat. Unlike the AAMC, AACOM does not regulate this part of the application process, and some of the osteopathic schools have become a little too aggressive, and in my mind, predatory in this regard. It's something I've tried to bring up directly with AACOM without much success.

Allopathic schools, on the other hand, do have some regulation of deposit amounts that each school can request. These deposits are also, oftentimes, refundable.

Be prepared to have up to $2500 dollars for a deposit to osteopathic schools and several hundred for allopathic schools.

Lost Opportunity Costs

Not often talked about are the opportunity costs of the application process—the money you aren't making at your job during the time you are at different stages of the application. If you work, you'll need to factor in the lost wages for days you may miss while studying for and taking the MCAT, traveling for interviews, and more. Not only do you have a lot of money going out, but you also will likely have less money coming in.

How to Afford the Application Cycle

The first step is to go to appexpenses.com to get a pretty good estimate on what you'll have to save to be financially ready for the medical school application costs.

Hopefully, you are reading this early enough in the cycle, or even before the cycle, that you can start to budget for the costs. If you estimate the cost of your application cycle will be around $4,000, and you have five months to save, you'll need to make sure you're putting away an extra $800 each month.

You might be able to look at how much you will need at each stage as well. Our expense calculator will give you that information, too. Maybe you will only need $800 for the primary application, which is three months away, then $1200 for secondaries, which are four months away, and $1000 for your interviews, which are likely still 5-6 months away.

If it's closer to the application cycle, and it will be hard to budget for the costs, you can look at getting a loan from your family, or even check out credit cards that offer an eighteen-month, 0% interest on purchases. The 0% interest credit cards are very popular for students to use during the application cycle. It's equivalent to having 18 months to budget, instead of four or five. However, you have to be very disciplined about paying off the credit card by the required date, or else all of that interest will be added to your balance.

We're adding more and more to appexpenses.com often, so please go check it out.

Application Cost Examples

It is hard for many students to actually understand the financial impact of the application cycle, just from talking about it. Let's look at an example for you to see what it may look like.

Let's assume some averages for our calculations here in the book.

The average number of applications a student submits through AMCAS is 17[2].

The average number of applications a student submits through AACOMAS is 9[3].

Let's assume a student is applying to both AMCAS and AACOMAS and applying to the average number of schools for each. That's 26 total schools. These estimates are based on current fees while writing this book and are subject to change. Text APPFEES to 44222 to see what current fees are.

- MCAT Self-Study Materials: $400
- MCAT Registration Fees: $320
- Transcript Fees: $20 (estimate for 2 schools)
- AMCAS Fees: $826 ($170 fee, which includes one school and $41 for the other 16 schools)
- AACOMAS Fees: $564 ($196 fee, which includes one school and $46 for the other eight schools)
- Secondary Fees: $1950 (based on an estimated average of $75 per school)
- CASPer Fees: $50 (estimate for sending to 4 schools plus the test fee)

We're already over $4,100, and we haven't had the chance to interview yet.

---

2   https://www.aamc.org/download/321442/data/factstablea1.pdf
3   https://www.aacom.org/docs/default-source/data-and-trends/2019-aacomas-applicant-pool-profile-summary-report.pdf

Let's assume you get three interview invites, and you go to all of them. Two of them are out of town, for which you'll need plane tickets and a hotel room for each. You'll also need transportation and food costs.

- New Suit: $300
- Airfare: $718 (based on the national average for ticket prices)
- Hotel: $516 (based on the national average for two nights at each interview)
- Transportation: $160 (based on $40 per day in ride-sharing costs)
- Food: $120 (based on $30 per day in food costs)

The month you are interviewing, you'll have to miss seven days of work—three days each for the out-of-town interviews, and one day for the in-town interview. Of course, you may be able to be strategic and fly after work the day before your interview and fly back very late the night of your interview, but I'd prefer, at least for your flight the day before, to plan to leave earlier in case your flight is canceled and you have to reschedule to a later flight. It's never a great phone call to the Admissions Committee when you planned a 9 pm flight that was canceled and the next one doesn't get in until mid-way through the interview day.

If you've applied to osteopathic medical schools, and your first acceptance is to one of those schools, let's assume you have to put down a $1,500 non-refundable deposit to hold your seat. If, later in the cycle, you are accepted to your local, state allopathic medical school (which was your first choice), you are now required to put down another deposit, and you'll forfeit the deposit to the osteopathic school.

You can see that the cost at the end of the day, assuming you get an acceptance, can be upwards of $6,000 to $7,000. When you factor in the opportunity cost of missed work and interest fees if you're not using a 0% interest card or cannot pay it off before the deadline, the true cost is much higher.

How are you supposed to pay for that if you're a working, single parent, or a starving student who doesn't have support from your parents?

I personally had a lot of credit card debt when I was younger. There were times when I owed thousands of dollars in a single month because of interest and other penalties. Fortunately, I've been able to fix that, but I understand the consequences of getting into too much credit card debt and not being able to pay those bills, so please be very careful.

If you are reading this book and you're preparing early enough, you can act as your own credit card and start saving every month. You can open up a high-interest checking account and deposit money into that account every month, depending on how many months you have until the application is due, and you need to start paying all of the application costs.

Scholarships

There are a lot of scholarships available to students—not specifically those applying to medical school, so please do a lot of research to see if you can apply for any of them and get some free money. We offer a scholarship that offers cash prizes at premedscholarship.com. A quick web search for "premed scholarships" returns a lot of options that may be able to help you.

Fee Assistance Program

The AAMC and AACOMAS both have fee-assistance programs (FAP) to help with the cost of applying to medical school. They each have their own specifics, and I encourage you to visit their websites for the most up-to-date information. TMDSAS does not offer a fee-assistance program because it is a single, flat-fee.

AAMC FAP

You are only eligible for the AAMC FAP if you are a citizen of the US, a US national, a Green Card holder, or a DACA student. You have to meet guidelines for poverty levels to qualify for the fee-assistance program. For example, for the AAMC FAP, if you have a family of four in California, your total family income has to be less than 300% of the national poverty level for that family size. In 2018, that amount was less than $75,300. You can go to the AAMC and AACOMAS websites to see their current guidelines.

When you are awarded the fee-assistance program from the AAMC, you also get access to the Medical School Admissions Requirements (MSAR), which helps you learn about the individual medical schools and their requirements.

You'll also get a reduced MCAT exam fee as well as free practice materials for the MCAT.

The AAMC FAP includes a waiver of all AMCAS fees with up to 20 schools that you designate in your application. The fee-assistance program information is typically transmitted to the medical schools and, if they wave their secondary fees for those with FAP, you should automatically have those fees waived.

You are allowed to earn FAP benefits from the AAMC five times.

For the AAMC, your benefits expire at the end of the calendar year after you received your award. For example, if you received your award on January 1, 2030, your fee-assistance program benefits will expire on December 31, 2031. If you apply prior to December 31, 2031, for the fee-assistance program again, and you again qualify, your initial fee-assistance program benefits will expire immediately, and your new benefits will kick in and expire the following calendar year.

AACOM FAP

To qualify for the fee-assistance program through AACOM, you need tax return information with income levels lower than 200% of the federal poverty guidelines. AACOM has a chart that lays out all of the information you need to see if you will qualify.

Unlike AAMC, which allows you to apply to 20 schools through their FAP, AACOMAS only waives the application fee, which includes the first school. You are still responsible for the additional fee for each additional program.

Because AACOM isn't affiliated with the MCAT, you don't get any of the MCAT benefits that the AAMC FAP offers you.

When you are awarded the FAP through AACOM, you must submit your AACOMAS application within 14 days. Because of this, you should only apply for it when you're very close to submitting your application.

Parental Financial Information

The fee-assistance program from the AAMC requires your parental financial information and supporting tax documentation. Their income is not added to yours, but they must also meet the eligibility guidelines for you to qualify for FAP. There is not an exemption for students who are nontraditional, married with kids, or if you haven't had a connection, especially financial, to your parents in 10 years.

There are opportunities to appeal this rule so you do not have to have your parent's information included in your application; however, if you ask people who go through this process, they will tell you it is a very time-consuming process that requires a lot of information.

For the AACOM FAP, if you were listed as a dependent on someone else's tax return, then you must provide their tax return instead of your own.

MCAT

The Medical College Admissions Test® (MCAT®) is administered by the AAMC, and has four sections on it:

- Chemical and Physical Foundations of Biological Sciences (Chem/Phys or C/P)
- Critical Analysis and Reasoning Skills (CARS)
- Biological and Biochemical Foundations of Living Systems (Bio/ Biochem or B/B)
- Psychological, Social and Biological Foundations of Behavior (Psych/ Soc or P/S)

The MCAT is over seven hours long and requires a lot of physical as well as mental stamina to make it through. If you didn't know, the MCAT is hard, and the MCAT is important. I have a primer to the MCAT that I published with Blueprint Prep, which can be found on Amazon by searching for *The Premed Playbook: Guide to the MCAT*.

While the MCAT is just one part of your application, it is a very big part. We'll discuss some of the most relevant topics in this book.

Your MCAT score is needed for your application to be considered complete by most schools. The score takes approximately one month to be released, and it is automatically transmitted to AMCAS schools. However, you'll have to release your score to AACOMAS and TMDSAS through the MCAT website.

You'll take the MCAT at a testing center where other students will be taking the MCAT or any number of other exams that the testing center administers. Depending on when you register, the testing center near you may not have any availability, and if you need to take the test on a specific date, you may have to travel to a testing center to take it.

Testing dates and locations typically open up for the beginning part of the year in October of the prior year. If you are planning to take the MCAT in March or April of 2030, you should start looking for dates beginning around October of 2029.

What is on the MCAT?

The AAMC doesn't hide what they will cover on the MCAT. They give rough estimates on the material so you can properly prepare.

Here are some breakdowns they provide:
- Chem/Phys:
  - First-semester biochemistry, 25%
  - Introductory biology, 5%
  - General chemistry, 30%
  - Organic chemistry, 15%
  - Introductory physics, 25%
- CARS:
  - Foundations of Comprehension, 30%
  - Reasoning Within the Text, 30%
  - Reasoning Beyond the Text, 40%
- Bio/Biochem:
  - First-semester biochemistry, 25%
  - Introductory biology, 65%

- General chemistry, 5%
- Organic chemistry, 5%
- Psych/Soc:
  - Introductory psychology, 65% (about 5% of this test section will include psychology questions that are biologically relevant. This is in addition to the discipline target of 5% for introductory biology)
  - Introductory sociology, 30%
  - Introductory biology, 5%

How Long is the MCAT?

The entire MCAT is about eight hours long. This includes an intro to the software, breaks, and lunch. There are 230 questions on the MCAT broken down into the following sections:

- Chemical and Physical Foundations of Biological Systems (59 items, 95 minutes)
- Critical Analysis and Reasoning Skills (53 items, 90 minutes)
- Biological and Biochemical Foundations of Living Systems (59 items, 95 minutes)
- Psychological, Social and Biological Foundations of Behavior (59 items, 95 minutes)

Since the MCAT is so long, one thing you need to do is prepare for it by practicing full-length exams. Sitting and staring at a screen for that long is exhausting, and you need to "train" for it. It's similar to someone training for a marathon by running really long distances all in one session. It would be very hard to train for a marathon, only doing one mile a day. This would be the equivalent of a student only doing question banks to prepare for the full MCAT. We'll talk about full-length exams later in the chapter.

When Should I Take the MCAT?

In a perfect world, you should take the MCAT no later than March of the year you are planning to apply to medical school. This will allow you to have your score back before you submit your application(s).

Depending on your specific situation, this timing may not be ideal. You may be finishing classes, hoping to get one final semester of a 4.0 under your belt before you apply. Many students are in this situation, which is what generally happens if they focus on classes before moving on to the other parts of the application. This is a huge mistake in my mind.

Let's say you finish classes in May. The next thing students do is study for the MCAT they scheduled for July. Because they are in a time-crunch to study for the MCAT, they ignore the application—personal statement, activities, asking for letters of recommendation, etc.

Once the student has taken their MCAT in July, assuming they didn't push it back, they will usually give themselves a little celebratory break before jumping into the applications. They will then start to work on the application and will rush it because they are already behind everyone else who submitted a couple of months ago already.

Remember, most medical schools operate on a rolling admissions basis, so your chances are usually better the earlier your applications are completed. This doesn't mean you should rush a bad application, but it does mean you need to think about the whole process and not just each individual part as you are preparing for your application.

How is the MCAT Scored?

The MCAT is composed of four different scores, one for each section. The scores range from 118 to 132, with the average being 125, or a 500 overall.

The MCAT is not scored on a curve. This is probably one of the biggest misconceptions of how it works. The AAMC states the MCAT is "scaled and equated." This means that when you take the test in February and score a 127 in one section, and another student takes the MCAT in April and also scores a 127 in that same section, medical schools can assume those scores are equal. Honestly, it's a little voodoo to me, but just trust that however your scoring is being handled is going to be the same for every other student.

One thing that does change year after year is the percentiles. Every year, the AAMC updates the MCAT percentiles to reflect the most recent three years of MCAT scoring data to show how well students compare to each other.

What is a Good MCAT Score?

This is the first question that premed students ask. They cut right to the chase and try to figure out what they need to do to get into medical school.

The most current data (2020-2021) from the AAMC shows the average MCAT score for those who matriculated into medical school was 511.5[4].

For students applying to DO schools through AACOMAS, the MCAT is much lower, averaging almost 504 according to the 2018 AACOMAS Profile report[5].

For TMDSAS matriculants, their MCAT scores are similar to the AAMC data.

You can see there is a big difference between the MCAT scores for those entering MD schools, either through TMDSAS or AMCAS, and DO schools through AACOMAS. That doesn't mean that DO schools are easier to get into—it just means, historically, that DO schools have valued diversity and nontraditional students more, and typically those students have had lower MCAT scores.

I am discovering more and more DO schools having higher MCAT targets for students, so I'm expecting the stats to come closer and closer together as time goes on.

If you can score higher than the averages above, then you can assume you've improved your chances of getting in. Lower than that, and you'll hurt your chances.

In an ideal world, you'll want to shoot for a 510 or above. Does that mean if you score a 508, you need to retake it? Absolutely not. A 508 is still a very good score.

If you are below 500, I would definitely recommend retaking the MCAT to make yourself more competitive. Again, that doesn't mean you *can't* get into medical school with a score below 500, but it makes it a lot harder.

I did a podcast interview on *The Premed Years* with Austin, a student who scored a 496 but was still able to get an interview and was accepted to medical school because other factors in his application stood out. You can listen to the interview in Session 335 of *The Premed Years* (premedyears.com/335).

---

4   https://www.aamc.org/media/6061/download (table A-17 for future years)

5   https://www.aacom.org/reports-programs-initiatives/aacom-reports/matriculants

Think of the MCAT as something that will either hurt or help your application and not the most important part of your application. Don't let online forums scare you into thinking you have to have a perfect MCAT score to get into medical school. You are much more than your stats.

Depending on what schools you are looking to get into and what part of the country you want to be in, you may or may not have to retake your MCAT exam based on your score. If you receive a 505 and you are applying broadly to MD and DO schools through AMCAS and AACOMAS, then I would say you likely have a decent shot of getting into medical school, assuming your GPA is also competitive, **and** you have a great story to tell in your application. If you're relying on stats alone and don't have good activities and a great story to tell, you may be out of luck.

If you are looking at going to Harvard, Washington University in St. Louis (WashU), or UCSF and you have a 505, then you might want to consider retaking the MCAT because those schools have very high standards and don't budge much on stats.

In various conversations with the Deans/Directors of Admissions of multiple medical schools, oftentimes it is not the Admissions Committee that sets these MCAT score standards, but rather pressure from the school boards to have the highest stats possible, with one school board saying that they wanted the **average** MCAT score for the matriculating class to be a 520.

Focusing on such vanity metrics doesn't do anyone justice, except the school's ego. It doesn't illustrate the quality of a class, curriculum, or education that you will receive at a particular institution.

My cutoff is typically 500. It's the general benchmark for most medical schools. If your score is less than a 500, I would retake it, no questions asked.

In *The Premed Years*, Session 328 (premedyears.com/328), I talked to Janet, who was a nontraditional student, a former nurse who scored 499 on her MCAT, and was told directly by an osteopathic medical school that they could not offer her an interview even though the rest of her application was great because she had less than a 500 MCAT score. Janet ultimately ended up getting two interviews and two acceptances to allopathic medical schools after advocating for herself at premed conferences.

What Score Do I Need if I Have a Low GPA?

Students often think that MCAT and GPA are on opposite ends of a scale, and if one is low, the other one needs to be high to "make up" for that. There is no sliding scale to tell you what you need to score based on your GPA, though. A high MCAT score helps everyone, so I don't think you can specifically say that a high MCAT score will help your low GPA. If your GPA is below a school's cutoff, they might still screen you out, even with a 520 MCAT.

Having a high MCAT score will give a medical school some comfort in your ability to do well in the classes and on the boards, and may help them overlook a less than stellar GPA. Whether your GPA is high or low, you should always be aiming as high as possible on the MCAT.

Do I Need to Worry about Sub-section Scores?

Every student has their own strengths and weaknesses. English as a second language (ESL) students tend to struggle with the CARS section. I've seen ESL students score 127+ in every section except for CARS, where they may have received a 122. The first question they ask is, "Is this going to hurt me?"

In Episode 1 of Mission Accepted (missionaccepted.tv), I interviewed a student who received an acceptance to school with a 121 on her CARS section. She had a 507, which included a 127 on Chem/Phys, 121 on CARS, 128 on Bio/Biochem, and a 130 on Psych/Soc.

As with everything, sub-section cutoffs are going to be school-dependent.

Can I Apply Without my MCAT?

You can submit your applications without an MCAT score. The verification processes for the application services do not require an MCAT score. Medical schools will see you are planning to take the MCAT, and most medical schools will put your application into an "incomplete pile" until your MCAT score is released before they will do a full review of your application to determine if they want to invite you for an interview.

During the COVID-19 pandemic, some schools accepted students without an MCAT score for the 2020-2021 application cycle; post-COVID, some schools might be thinking about routes to an acceptance without an MCAT score, but that is yet to be determined.

Should I Apply with a (Really) Low Score?

If you received your MCAT score and you're ashamed of it, don't be. It's okay. A low MCAT score doesn't mean anything. Whether your score is borderline or terrible, your retake is what is going to be the biggest determining factor in getting into medical school. Medical schools will not look at your initial score and assume you aren't cut out for medical school based on that one score. Instead, they will wait until your retake comes back to determine your competency for medical school and determine if they want to invite you for an interview.

In *The Premed Years*, Session 422 (premedyears.com/422), Michael shared his story of being a 5x MCAT tester and 5x applicant to medical school. With only one interview invite over his first four cycles, and a maximum MCAT score of 506, he finally nailed the MCAT with a 515 for his 5th cycle and had nine interview invites. The schools didn't care about his previous terrible scores, just that he showed improvement in his activities, MCAT score, and GPA through a master's program.

If you think you'll have a competitive MCAT score released before September of the application year, then I would suggest you still submit your application. If you really struggled with the MCAT and it's going to take you a while to improve your score, don't submit the application, or don't fill out any secondaries if you did submit. Don't waste any more money on the current cycle, and take your time preparing properly for the MCAT. Plan to move to the next application cycle.

If you do think you'll be ready to take the MCAT and get a more competitive score, one thing you can do is add only one school to your application for AMCAS and AACOMAS, so you don't have to pay the individual school fees. Your application can be submitted, and you can start the verification process. When you get your score back, if it's where you need it to be, then you can add more schools to your list. If you do this, you may want to start prewriting secondaries for the schools you will likely add to your list if you receive a good score. Once you add more schools, you'll get secondary requests from those new schools pretty quickly.

When you submit with just one school, you're getting your application verified as soon as possible. Many students wait, and it can cause massive delays in the verification processing, especially through AMCAS since it has historically been very slow with verification times.

Waiting for Your Score to Apply

If you wait to submit your application until your MCAT score is back, you jeopardize your whole application, even if the rest of it is good.

If you take the MCAT at the end of June and you don't submit your application until the end of July when your score is released, your application, through AMCAS, likely won't be verified and ready to be reviewed until the end of August, at the earliest. You will likely still get secondary essays from the schools before your application is verified, and you can start submitting those as soon as possible. Your application will be complete by the end of August or the beginning of September, assuming you can turn around all of the secondary essays quickly. While this isn't "horrible," you should plan for something earlier.

If you submitted your application to one school at the end of June when you took the MCAT, then started working on secondaries and turned them around quickly, your application would theoretically be complete almost a month before. Since most medical schools use rolling admissions, a month is a very long delay and can be the difference between an interview and a rejection.

Is it Bad to Retake the MCAT?

Medical schools know the MCAT is hard. It's common for students to need to take the MCAT more than once. If you are one of those students, it's okay. Good students do poorly on the MCAT because they go into it thinking it's just another test when it is not. The preparation for the MCAT is very different than any other test you have taken as an undergraduate student, which is oftentimes reflected in your first MCAT score.

What looks bad is having multiple scores showing you are taking the MCAT too soon and getting the same score or worse. Seeing a trend of an MCAT score of 500, and then having a 499 a month later, shows the Admissions Committee you are impulsive and not able to reflect on your study habits to properly prepare for the MCAT. It may raise concerns for them.

If you take the MCAT the first time and aren't prepared for the difficulty of the exam and you score a 490, but you retake the exam and you score a 498, that shows you've done a lot to improve your score. And if you can come back and then score a 502 or 505, you've shown even more growth for the MCAT. Just like an upward trend in GPA, that trend for your MCAT score is very telling of the type of student you can be.

How Do Schools View Multiple MCAT Scores?

Every medical school is going to look at multiple MCAT scores differently. Some schools may use what is known as a super score. This is very common in the SAT world in which undergraduate institutions take your highest scores from every section of the test and add those together for your composite score. Some medical schools will do this with your MCAT, though it is not very common.

Some schools will look at your highest MCAT score. Some schools will look at your most recent MCAT score. Ultimately, you have no control over how a medical school is going to view multiple MCAT scores, so it is not something you should be wasting your time trying to figure out. Do your best on the MCAT and apply with a solid application—don't think you can game the system by finding the schools that are going to work best for your MCAT score.

I don't think it is wise to call medical schools to ask them how they review multiple MCAT scores. If you have multiple MCAT scores, then you will need to apply broadly and hope the rest of your application is strong as well.

How Many Times Can I Take the MCAT?

Over the life of your MCAT test-taking, you can sit for it up to seven times. Obviously, I hope that none of you have to take it seven times, but that is the maximum you are allowed. There are also limits to how many times you can take it within a calendar year and within a two-year period.

Ultimately, the MCAT is just one part of your application. A low MCAT score doesn't necessarily ruin your chances of getting into medical school. If you can't seem to get a good MCAT score no matter what you do, there are other options out there, including going to the Caribbean.

In the End, It Doesn't Matter

Remember, once you are a doctor, your patients will never ask you what you got on your MCAT. A low MCAT score does not mean you will not be a good doctor. It does not mean you can't be a doctor. It just means you got a low MCAT score.

#respectthemcat

When you're on social media talking about the MCAT and being premed, start using #respectthemcat. It's time we get other students to realize how hard of a test it is.

GPA

Before I even start this chapter, I need to make it known that AMCAS, AACOMAS, and TMDSAS all have their own ways of calculating a student's GPA and determining what courses actually need to be included. Everything I'm about to tell you may reflect one application service, two of them, or all of them. Please read each application service's instruction manual before starting this process.

The moment you step foot on a college campus, whether it's a trade school, community college, or a four-year university, everything you do can either hurt or help your medical school application. Even as a high school student taking dual-enrollment courses, the decisions you make while still a "kid" can severely derail your path to getting into medical school.

If you have courses from an international school and you transfer those classes to a US school to count towards your degree, you may have to report those courses as well. I've seen many students think they could "run away" from their poor academic performance in another country and start fresh here, only to make the mistake of transferring in those classes and having those poor grades haunt them in the future as well.

Your GPA is a full picture of your academic record. Every class you've taken, and every class you've failed. Every class you've retaken, and every class you've aced. They all count. There is no "hiding" when it comes to your coursework. Every blemish will be seen.

One of the biggest mistakes students make when starting undergrad is taking on too much, too fast, and they end up stretching themselves too thin. This is especially true for freshmen premeds, who hit the ground running during their first college semester, straight into a full, difficult course load of hard sciences while also joining every premed club on campus and volunteering in the hospital. It can be hard to recover after starting off poorly, but it's doable, assuming the student still has the motivation and confidence to do it.

How are GPAs Calculated?

For almost everyone reading this book, every class you've ever taken for college credit, even if you stepped foot in the class for one day and later withdrew, needs to be accounted for on your application. Even if your school replaces or removes repeated classes, you need to enter those original classes on your application, as they will still count in the GPA calculation. You may ask yourself, "If the class isn't on my application, how are they ever going to know I failed it?" If you're asking yourself that, stop. If you go down this path of falsifying your application and it is discovered, you can kiss your career goodbye.

The GPA you see on your school's transcript will almost certainly not be the same one that the medical schools will see.

The general guideline for grades is as follows:

- A or A+ = 4.0
- A- = 3.7 (4.0 for TMDSAS)
- B+ = 3.3 (3.0 for TMDSAS)
- B = 3.0
- B- = 2.7 (3.0 for TMDSAS)
- C+ = 2.3 (2.0 for TMDSAS)
- C = 2.0

- C- = 1.7 (2.0 for TMDSAS)
- and so on.

AMCAS

AMCAS will convert the grades provided by your institution to a standard format so students who went to schools with different grading structures or different academic systems (think semesters vs. quarters) can all be compared on a level playing field.

If your school has a different grading system (i.e., numbers vs. letters, or AB vs. A- or B+), AMCAS provides a conversion table that you can easily search for using the term "AMCAS Grade Conversion Chart."

BCPM vs. AO

For the AMCAS application, your science GPA consists of Biology, Chemistry, Physics, and Math courses (BCPM). Classes that are not classified as BCPM are known as AO, or "All Other." It is up to you, as you are entering your courses into the application, to classify the courses correctly.

You can search the web for "AMCAS Course Classification Guide" to get the latest information from AMCAS to assist you in classifying your classes properly. If you misclassify a course or two, AMCAS will usually correct it. If you have a lot of errors in the classification of your courses, AMCAS will send your application back to you to fix, which will delay your verification process.

PDF Breakdowns

When you print your application in PDF form, your AMCAS grades are calculated on a per-year and overall basis. If you have graduate coursework, this is all calculated under a "Graduate" heading. Undergraduate postbac work is classified under a "Postbaccalaureate Undergraduate" heading, but it is also calculated into your cumulative undergraduate GPA.

AACOMAS

The major difference between AMCAS and AACOMAS is the calculation of your science and "all other" GPA. AACOMAS does not consider math as a science course and therefore only calculates your science GPA based on your BCP courses. This can be helpful for students who struggled with math. However, those math classes are still calculated into your overall GPA and your "non-science GPA."

PDF Breakdowns

When you print your application in PDF form, AACOMAS calculates a lot of different GPAs that you can see when you print out your application. It will break down every type of subject matter, different years, overall, etc. Medical schools will use this however they want when determining who they want to invite for an interview.

TMDSAS

The biggest difference between TMDSAS and AMCAS is the fact that TMDSAS does not use +/- grades to calculate your GPA. Thus, receiving a B+ is calculated the same as a B-.

Science GPAs are calculated similarly to AMCAS with a BCPM scoring system.

PDF Breakdowns

When you print your application in PDF form, TMDSAS calculates eight GPAs for your application: overall GPA, overall BCPM, overall undergraduate, undergraduate BCPM, undergraduate non-BCPM, overall graduate, graduate BCPM, and graduate non-BCPM GPA.

A Note on PDF Breakdowns

I want to make one important clarification on the GPA calculations that you see versus what the medical schools see. Every piece of data you enter into your application will go to the medical school. Each medical school uses software that they have licensed to evaluate and view the data exactly how they want to view it. AMCAS may show you a grid of GPA data based on year and science (BCPM) vs. non-science (AO), but the medical school may break it down into a dozen more slices to evaluate your performance.

Is My GPA Good Enough?

That is the question many of you are thinking about right now. It is such a hard question to answer because your 3.2 GPA differs from your roommate's 3.2 GPA. Your roommate might have a 3.2 every semester of their academic career. You, on the other hand, started off pretty poorly adjusting in your undergrad and had a very poor GPA early on, but then you turned it around and, for the last two years, have a 4.0 GPA.

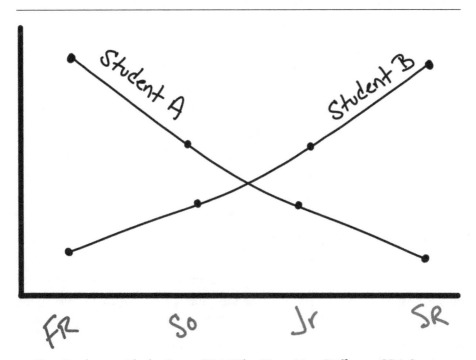

Two Students with the Same GPA Who Have Very Different GPA Stories

It's impossible to look at just your current or final GPA and get a picture of who you are as a student. I can't tell you whether or not you are ready to apply based on just your GPA or potentially how competitive you are as an applicant. Whenever students come to me and ask for help leading with their GPA, the first thing I have them do is calculate their GPA and trends. I have a GPA calculator on the website that you can use at whatsmygpa.com.

Ideally, to get past the "digital shredders" and be considered for an interview, you should have a GPA higher than 3.0 for both your science GPA and overall GPA. The lower your GPA, the longer (i.e., more credits) your trend needs to be.

Does My Science GPA Matter More?

Your overall GPA and science GPA both matter. I know it's not the answer that you want to hear, but it is true—your overall academic record matters. Obviously, a science GPA shows medical schools that you are academically competent for science courses. That is important and why sciences are so heavily tested when it comes to being a premed.

Some of you may be nontraditional students with a poor academic record from undergrad in a business degree or some other liberal arts degree. That is actually great for you because as you are coming back and taking courses in a postbac program, you have the ability to earn a really strong science GPA. As long as your cumulative GPA doesn't filter you out from medical schools, you'll still have a very good shot at getting into medical school, even with a lower overall GPA.

Remember that the goal for both MCAT and GPA (outside of being a perfect 528 and 4.0 student) is to have good enough stats to make it through the filters and to be high enough in the stack of applications that a school is going to have the opportunity to review your application before they run out of interview spots. The interview spots are the limiting factor when it comes to the application process. Medical schools only have so many interview spots to give out every year, and once those are gone, they are gone, and no other students can be evaluated for an interview.

How Can I Improve My GPA?

A lot of students don't understand what steps can be taken to improve their GPA. A great deal of you may have been told or may believe that once your GPA is "final"—once you are done with college—there are no other opportunities to improve your GPA, especially your undergraduate GPA.

You probably know you can go on and get a master's degree, and many of you have done that, but did you know you can also just continue to take classes at an undergraduate institution, whether it's your own or a different one, or even at a community college? Taking classes after you graduate from college is known as a postbac (short for postbaccalaureate). Your undergraduate degree is known as a baccalaureate degree, and so a postbac is taking undergraduate classes after already receiving your baccalaureate degree.

Do-It-Yourself Postbacs

There are many ways to take postbac classes. You can go to the same school you went to as an undergrad and just continue to register for classes. Some schools may let you register as a non-degree-seeking student, meaning you're not looking to get another degree. Some schools will require you to declare another major and state you are going to complete another degree.

When you are registering for courses outside of a formal postbac program, you are doing what is known as a "do-it-yourself," or DIY, postbac.

In the end, it doesn't matter if you have to declare another degree because you can drop out, just like many other students do every semester. Take the classes you need to improve your GPA and when you are done, just stop going and stop registering for classes. The second degree makes no difference when it comes to applying to medical school—it's only the extra classes for your GPA that matter.

Community College

If you need to work to put food on the table and a roof over your head, you may find that community college courses have a better schedule that fits your working life. Taking postbac classes at a community college is okay. Not every medical school will like it, but if that is what you need to do, then you will find a way to make it work. Be prepared to talk about why you went to community college in your interviews. Beyond that, don't worry or upend your life to avoid taking postbac classes at a community college.

I had a great interview with David on *The Premed Years* about his journey as a dad and full-time software engineer while also going to school at a community college to complete his prereqs. He had plenty of interviews and great acceptances to choose from, but he did have to talk about why he did so much work at a community college. You can listen to that interview at premedyears.com/330.

Formal Postbacs

There are formal postbac programs out there that are ready and willing to take your money in exchange for a lot more structure and access to advising that you may not get at a do-it-yourself postbac. Columbia was the first postbac program here in the United States, offering a place for soldiers after the war to come back and get more education to transition them into their next career. Postbac programs can be very expensive to attend, and depending on the financial aid situation, you may or may not be able to get financial aid for them.

There are two different types of postbac programs. There are "career-changer" postbac programs for students who have very little to no science courses. This would be for someone who majored in English or who was out in the business world and now wants to be a physician and needs to start taking general chemistry and complete all of their science courses. There are also "academic enhancer" programs for the student who may have been premed or may have been in another science program or science major but didn't do well and needs to take a lot of the courses over again to prove their academic competence. If you have only a few science courses, reach out to some of the career-changer programs to see if you can still apply.

Some of these postbac programs require an MCAT score, while others do not. I personally don't understand why the postbac programs require an MCAT score when the goal in the postbac program is to improve your foundational science knowledge so that, hopefully, you can do well on the MCAT.

Master's Programs

If you are looking to do a master's program, make sure it is something that is more hard-science-heavy. You can get a master's in chemistry, biology, or in a lot of other heavy sciences.

If you are struggling with your science courses and you need to prove your science competency to medical schools, getting a Master of Public Health will not help you in that regard. It may give you access to the school or to the faculty, but it's not going to assure medical schools that you can handle the academic rigors of medical school.

A lot of students look at master's programs above everything else because of the ability to get financial aid.

Special Master's Program

A Special Master's Program (SMP) is basically a master's level postbac program. They are usually specifically designed for pre-health students, and oftentimes their students take classes with first-year medical students. Many SMPs are situated on-campus with a medical school, and it can be a good audition for medical school, assuming all goes well. It can be your last shot at proving to the medical school that you can handle the curriculum because you're sitting in the same classroom as first-year medical students taking the same classes and the same tests. If you can do well in an SMP, you are assuring the medical school you will do well as a medical school student. Like formal postbac programs, you may or may not be able to get financial aid to go to an SMP, and they can be fairly expensive.

Should I Do a Master's Program or an Undergrad Postbac?

At the end of the day, from what I've seen and understood, from talking to Admissions Committee members, like Dr. Scott Wright, the former Director of Admissions at UT Southwestern, my co-host on Ask the Dean, and the VP of Academic Advising at Mappd, and from talking to students going through this process every year, it seems that undergraduate grades are more heavily weighted when it comes to the application process. If you have a 2.8 undergraduate GPA and a 3.7 graduate GPA, your 2.8 undergraduate GPA may still hold you back from a lot of schools.

Don't take this to mean that you can't get into medical school if the only viable next step for you is a master's level program instead of an undergraduate postbac program. I had two great interviews with students on *The Premed Years* podcast concerning this topic. Nneka (premedyears.com/261) had a 2.7 GPA from Cornell and had to do a master's program that worked with her schedule.

Sabina (premedyears.com/385) is another student who struggled in her undergrad, completed a master's program, and is now excelling in medical school.

If all things were equal and you had no limitations with finances or your schedule, my recommendation would be to do an undergrad postbac. It does not matter if it is a do-it-yourself postbac where you're just taking classes on your own or a postbac that includes the advising structure and class structure of a formal program.

The goal depends on your starting point. If you're a strong student who needs science courses, your goal is to continue to be a strong student. If your goal is to show improved grades and a strong upward trend in your GPA, your goal is to become a strong student. You may never get your cumulative or science GPA above a 3.0, but if you can get upwards of 30-45 credits close to a 4.0, you are likely going to ease the concerns of the medical school. Remember, the goal is to prove to the admissions committees that your academic struggles are a thing of the past, that you have learned how to be a good student, and that you are ready for medical school.

Many students don't like that response because they think having a higher GPA in a master's program is "more impressive" than barely getting above a 3.0 for an undergrad GPA. One thing missing from that discussion is your GPA trend. Yes, your overall GPA may not look amazing at a glance, but once a medical school can give your application a more holistic evaluation, they will be able to see the trend in your grades. There is also some concern that most students do well in master's programs, so it may not have as much of an impact.

How Do Medical Schools Look at GPA?

When medical schools pull down your application, they do not specifically see what you see when you print out your application. As I mentioned above, they can sort and manipulate the data to make sure they are viewing applications how they want.

Some medical schools will only look at the last 20 hours of your science classes to determine if you will be academically ready for medical school. You could have a 3.0 GPA overall, but if your last 20 hours of science courses are a 4.0, that school sees you as a 4.0 student. Some schools, like the University of Illinois, have the ability to erase a year's worth of your grades. If you went through a bad breakup or a death in the family during sophomore year, those grades can be filtered out, and a new GPA can be calculated for you, and that is the GPA the school will judge you on. Dr. Leila Amiri talked about this on *The Premed Years* Session 288 (premedyears.com/288).

There's also something known as the 32-hour rule, which some medical schools have, most prominently LSU. The 32-hour rule states if you have struggled early on with your academics, but you take 32 hours of additional courses, the last 32 hours of your courses will be calculated as your GPA.

Texas has a program for its residents known as Academic Fresh Start. If you have college courses from over ten years ago, you can enroll in college for another degree, and your previous courses are cleared from your academic record. Only Texas medical schools and TMDSAS recognize this program. It's a great program for nontraditional Texans. The medical schools don't see your original grades, only that you were a Fresh Start Student.

What you need to understand is the majority of medical schools out there understand that you are human. They understand that life happens—breakups, deaths, and illnesses occur—and they are willing to be flexible because of that. If you find a medical school that won't cut you any slack because your parent died sophomore year and you received a bunch of bad grades, and they won't give you the benefit of the doubt even though you came back with amazing stats, you don't want to go to that school anyway. What happens when you struggle as a medical student at that school? They are probably not going to cut you any slack there, either. You want to find schools that understand you are human and you are not perfect. The far majority of medical schools out there will see you as that.

So, if you've gone through this journey and you have struggled at some point in your academic career, or you've been told by an adviser or a mentor that that one "C" or bad semester means you can no longer get into medical school, they are wrong. No matter what has happened with your academic past, you can overcome this and show the medical schools that you can handle what is going to come.

Should I apply with the GPA I Have?

This is the ultimate question asked by every student with a borderline or low GPA. The answer is simple—it depends. If you think your application is strong outside of a lower total (science and/or cumulative) GPA, then I would potentially pull the trigger and apply and let the medical schools tell you no. If your adviser is telling you not to apply because your GPA is low, I would listen to them with a grain of salt and determine for yourself if it is what you want to do.

What is considered low? If you have a 2.6 GPA with no upward trend or potentially a downward trend, your GPA is not low, your GPA is really bad. A low GPA, for this discussion, is something around a 3.1 or a 3.2, with a positive upward trend, at least for a little bit. I would pull the trigger and let the medical schools look at your application and let you know if you are competitive enough. They may come back and tell you no, that you need to take some more courses to show more of an upward trend, but let them tell you that. Let it come directly from the horse's mouth.

Now, I know you may be thinking that if you've finished your undergrad degree and you're taking more courses, the denominator in the GPA calculation is so big that the GPA needle doesn't move much—that is true. You may apply one year with a 3.2, not get in, and be told you need to show more academic rigor, but the next year you apply with a 3.23 after receiving all straight "A"s in that time period. It's a very different picture, however, even with a similar GPA. That's why you can't compare your overall number to anyone else because you don't know what is making up their GPA calculation.

At the end of the day, if you have a low GPA, you will have to determine if it is right for you to apply to medical school now or after some grade repair. You can sign up for a free two-week trial of Mappd and enter your courses to calculate your GPA and look at the trends to determine what you should do.

SECTION I

PRIMARY APPLICATION

TRANSCRIPTS

One of the most common questions I see in our Facebook Group (Premed Hangout) is whether or not you need to request transcripts from a particular school. The answer is almost always yes. If you have a complicated college journey, with lots of colleges, or overseas trips, or even attendance from a foreign institution, you must read the application instructions and find out what you have to do. This is one part of the instruction manual that I try to read every year because it has always been confusing to me, especially foreign transcripts.

The basic rule of thumb is this: if you were a student—submit the transcript. This includes dual enrollment while in high school, EMT license courses, military education, and other vocational or paraprofessional courses. Even if the course you took was not at a traditional school, you may need to submit a transcript. Read the instruction manual and contact the application help desk if you need further clarification.

You also need a transcript if you stepped foot in class for one day, withdrew, and never showed up again. Remember, if you are unsure if you need a transcript, the answer is likely yes. Again, please read the instruction manual and contact the application help desk if you need further clarification.

How to Request Transcripts

You'll need to print out the transcript request form from the application service **after** the application cycle opens for the year in which you are planning on applying. You'll need to follow your school's policies for requesting transcripts, including paying any fees associated with sending them.

For AMCAS and AACOMAS, after you add the schools that you've attended to the application service, you can then print a custom transcript request form for each of those schools. For TMDSAS, you can print out a generic transcript request form that has your TMDSAS ID pre-populated.

Transcripts are sent to each of the application services directly. Depending on your institution, they may be sent electronically or physically mailed. This does not matter; as long as the application service gets them, you will be set. Each service has a different way to verify if your transcripts have been received, so keep an eye on those notifications if you are starting to worry something got lost.

You do not need to send transcripts to schools. An exception to this might be if you are updating medical schools about completed coursework that you took after you submitted your application.

When to Request Transcripts

The application cycle timeline coincides perfectly with the academic calendar, and many students are just wrapping up a block of classes as they are getting ready to submit their applications. Don't get bombarded with whether or not you should wait until grades come out to submit your application.

According to the TMDSAS Application Handbook, your Spring grades must be on your transcript unless you're in a quarter system school, in which case you'll need your most recent Winter grades. There are some other exceptions, which you'll find in the Application Handbook.

For AMCAS and AACOMAS, if waiting for your Spring grades is going to significantly impact your ability to be verified early, I wouldn't wait. The only exception would be if you really *need* those grades to show an upward trend in your GPA (more on upward trends later).

While the application services need your transcript to verify your application, you do not need the finalized Spring semester grades to be on them before you submit. You can request your finalized transcripts after you submit your application, as the application service will wait for your transcripts before reviewing and verifying your application. The one drawback to this is if something changes after you submit. Your application may get kicked back to you for correction, which will delay the whole process even longer than if you had waited for the official transcripts.

EARLY DECISION PROGRAMS

Early decision programs (EDP) are an application process in which you apply to only one school, and if you are accepted, you must go to that school. You cannot apply EDP to one school through each application service—you must only apply to one medical school. If you have always dreamed about going to your local state medical school, and they allow EDP applications, then you should apply; hopefully, you'll get an interview, and you'll know, historically by the end of September, if you have been accepted.

At first glance, EDP seems like it's a no-brainer. Apply to only one school, get an interview, get an acceptance, and go on vacation until medical school starts. Even TMDSAS has the following on their website, "By applying for Early Decision you can greatly reduce the high financial and psychological costs of applying to and interviewing at multiple schools." Who wouldn't want to greatly reduce the high financial and psychological costs? Unfortunately, it's not that easy. Applying EDP is difficult and carries risks. Let's talk about some basics first.

The EDP application timeline is very similar to the normal application timeline. EDP is administered through the normal application services, but the deadlines are shifted forward. If you are going to apply EDP, you should check what the deadlines are for the school and application service to which you are going to apply.

Not every medical school participates in EDP, so you'll have to do some research for a current list of schools that participate.

Why It's Risky

Applying Early Decision requires that you not apply to any other medical schools. If you apply Early Decision through AMCAS, you are contractually saying you will not apply to any TMDSAS schools or any AACOMAS schools, either. One school. One decision. The timing of that decision is the key to why it is risky to apply Early Decision.

The date for knowing if you've been accepted or rejected can be as late as October 15th. If you are not accepted through EDP, you then can enter the regular applicant pool if you still wish to be considered by other medical schools. Remember, the other applicants who didn't apply EDP, yet who might have applied early after applications open, are already interviewing and receiving acceptances by that point.

By applying Early Decision and not getting accepted, you're potentially four months behind other applicants. Getting notified on October 1st and having to enter the regular applicant pool makes your application significantly late for other schools. If you're a strong applicant, you still have a chance to get in, but it makes your job a lot harder.

That is the biggest risk of Early Decision—being late.

Applying Early Decision should be done very cautiously if it is what you want to do. I would highly recommend you start building a relationship with the Admissions Committee, and specifically with the Dean/Director of Admissions if you can. Let them know you are thinking about applying Early Decision to their program. Lay out why you want to apply Early Decision and have them look at your application, if they will. Because the Early Decision program is a unique application program, many medical schools are happy to talk to students who are interested in applying for it. Some even may request that you do so before you apply.

Other Thoughts on EDP

It was very hard to find specific stats for Early Decision programs. There is not a lot of data to let you know, one way or another, what you should do. What is clear is that if you are rejected, you are a late applicant, and that is a big risk.

Something else to think about is financial aid. If you are an applicant to a medical school in the regular application pool, schools may use financial aid packages to help entice you to go to their school. If they really like you and want you, they can throw some money at you to help you make your decision.

As an Early Decision applicant, you are only applying to one school, and you are telling that medical school that you only want to go there, so they don't have to woo you with financial aid.

Applying Early Decision in and of itself does not increase your chances of getting into that medical school. You still need to be a good fit for that school. You still need to have good stats for that school. As I couldn't find great stats, I won't tell you if applying EDP makes it more or less competitive for that school. I'm just focusing on the risks.

Should I Apply EDP?

If you do a search and try to look for Early Decision information, you will see that it seems like the majority of people do not recommend Early Decision for students. At the end of the day, for over 95 percent of the students I talk to, I do not recommend Early Decision for them. I believe the risks outweigh the benefits.

If you are significantly tied to a specific area, and it will be hard for you to move, Early Decision may be the right move for you. For instance, if you are a mom with kids integrated into that community and a spouse with a specific job that is hard to relocate, you may not want to uproot your family so you can go to medical school. While applying Early Decision may be a good idea for you, remember that applying Early Decision doesn't negate the need for strong stats. You may actually need better stats.

I don't think Early Decision is right for students who just want to stay close to home without any other reasons. Early decision is not for someone who loved their undergrad experience and wants to continue at the same campus or school.

Application and Interview Timing

Here is one scenario in which you might want to throw your hat in the ring for one cycle of EDP. One student I was working with fell into this category. If you have a job that requires you to be outside of the country starting in October, with no chance to return for interviews, I wouldn't recommend applying to medical school for the current cycle because if you can't make it back for interviews, that's not going to work very well. Most medical schools will not allow you to interview virtually (this was written pre-COVID; it is yet to be seen if schools will be more flexible with virtual interviews in the future). If this is a situation you may be in, why not apply Early Decision? Assuming your stats are good enough, why not apply Early Decision to one school, assuming you have strong ties to it? If you're invited for an interview, it will happen before you have to leave. If med schools, post-COVID, are more flexible with virtual interviews on a case-by-case basis, this may not matter as much, and I would probably recommend staying away from EDP for this specific scenario.

If you can think of other scenarios that might make it reasonable for you to apply Early Decision, then go for it.

Mitigating Risks

Just remember the risks and try to do everything possible to mitigate those risks. While you are waiting for your decision, assume you are not going to get in and start building, if you haven't already, a school list of other medical schools you will want to apply to after being notified by your EDP school.

You should start prewriting secondaries for those schools. As soon as you can, you can add more schools to your school list. You will likely get secondary requests for those schools within a couple of days. The sooner you can turn around those secondaries, the better your chances are at mitigating a later application.

DISADVANTAGED STATUS ESSAY

There is no one path to medical school. Some premeds are children of physicians, and others are children of immigrant farmworkers making a minimum wage who rely on government assistance. No matter where you are from, if you have gotten to this point, you have shown the world that you are ready to tackle *anything*.

If you come from an upbringing that didn't afford you the same potential opportunities as the average student, marking yourself as disadvantaged in the AMCAS application will allow you to explain yourself. What if your upbringing was okay, but now, as a nontraditional student, you are in a disadvantaged situation? AMCAS does not define who should mark themselves as disadvantaged. If you feel like you are, say yes and explain yourself.

AACOMAS and TMDSAS do not give you the ability to mark yourself as disadvantaged.

Marking yourself as disadvantaged doesn't mean you have to have bad grades or a bad MCAT score. On the contrary, if you have a story to tell about your disadvantage, and you're able to show that you still performed well in school and on the MCAT despite your disadvantage, that shows the schools even more about you.

The specific question that AMCAS is asking you to answer is, "Do you wish to be considered a disadvantaged applicant by any of your designated medical schools that may consider such factors (social, economic, or educational)?" This question is intentionally vague to allow you to determine what it means for your life and your upbringing.

In your AMCAS application, the Disadvantaged Status question is in the Biographic Information tab. When you check "Yes," AMCAS allows you to write a 1,325 character length essay with the following prompt: "Please use the space to explain why you believe you should be considered a disadvantaged applicant by your designated medical schools."

Who Should Mark Yes?

AMCAS gives you some rough guidelines on what it means to be a disadvantaged applicant. One that most students get caught up in is the definition.

Every one of you reading this right now thinking about marking yourself as disadvantaged likely has a million questions running through your head. "What about this?" "What about that?" I could triple the size of this book with every possible scenario, and you would still have a unique scenario you would want to be answered.

Remember, AMCAS leaves the question and guidelines vague for a reason. If you feel like you are at a disadvantage, mark yourself as disadvantaged and write your essay. We will talk about some of the consequences of marking yourself disadvantaged and not explaining yourself well later.

Here are the AMCAS guidelines as of the time of the writing of this book:

1) Underserved: If you are from an underserved area, your exposure to medicine and healthcare may have started later than others, giving you potentially less time to explore the field and less networking ability to talk to those in the field already.

2) Immediate Family: Family issues are hard. They are your family, and you are supposed to love them and stick by them. Sometimes doing that means your

educational pursuits need to be put on hold, or they are wiped out altogether. If you feel like a situation with an immediate family member has hindered you and your pursuit of being a physician, you should mark "Yes."

3) State and Federal Assistance Programs: Mark "Yes" to the Disadvantaged Status question if you or your family has been on any state or federal assistance programs for any reason.

These are just three examples that AMCAS provides to students, but there are many other reasons you may want to tell your story.

I know a student who came to the US at the age of 18 to go to college. His parents were financially supporting him, but they didn't come to the US. He came with his sister, who was several years younger than he was, and he was her support system. Thousands of miles away from his family, being a "parent" to his sister, learning a new culture and language, and also being a college student all at the same time would be an incredible burden for anyone. Even though he had an amazing GPA and a great MCAT score, I advised him to mark himself as disadvantaged.

If you grew up on the South Side of Chicago and had to avoid gang activity to get to and from school every day, you *could* mark yourself as disadvantaged, even if you're not in an underserved area, were on assistance programs, or had any other family issues.

If you are a survivor of domestic abuse, a veteran struggling with PTSD, have had to work since the age of 12 to support your single mom, or have been homeless at any point in your life, you *can* mark yourself as disadvantaged.

Being from a marginalized group does not automatically make you disadvantaged, but how it has affected you may make you disadvantaged. I shared this chapter with many students before publishing this book, and no matter how many examples I put in here, someone will still ask, "But what about…"

If you are questioning if **you** could be considered disadvantaged based on your specific situation, the answer is yes. What I want you to do now is stop wondering *if* you can say yes and start thinking about *why* you want to say yes.

The most important part of the Disadvantaged Status essay is reflecting on *why* and *how* the experiences you're telling the Admissions Committee have affected you. This will give context to your entire application and may move you from a "maybe" to a "YES."

Who Should Not Mark Yes?

It is not up to me, or AMCAS, or your advisor to determine if your specific situation is a disadvantage or not. That's not to say there are not bad reasons why students mark themselves as disadvantaged. If you grew up in a wealthy neighborhood and you only had one butler instead of three like your friends, that is not a disadvantage.

If you are a first-generation college student, that usually isn't enough in my mind to say you were disadvantaged. Not having a parent help you navigate the college world doesn't keep you from going to advisors or professors for the same help. You should not play the "what if" game in your essay. "If my parents had college degrees, they could have helped me when I was struggling in my freshman year" is not a reason to mark yourself as disadvantaged.

If you are a first-generation college student who was often left at home alone because your parents both worked two jobs and you raised your younger sibling, then you may want to mark yourself as disadvantaged. Needing to be the "parent" affects the time you have to be a kid, to learn, and to take advantage of the same educational opportunities as your peers. Even if you have amazing stats, if you are from this type of background, marking yourself as disadvantaged and telling your story shows what you have been able to accomplish with what many would consider fewer opportunities.

How Does Marking Yourself as Disadvantaged Affect Your Application?

Every medical school has its own process for reviewing applications. This includes how they review the Disadvantaged Status essay. It's impossible to know if they may "boost" your GPA a little bit because of your situation. You can't guess if they may ignore your lower MCAT score because of your disadvantaged essay.

How each medical school, Admissions Committee, and reviewer views and weighs your disadvantaged essays is going to be different everywhere. This should not dissuade you from marking yourself as disadvantaged.

Even without knowing how your application will be affected, if you feel like your path was disadvantaged in any way, mark yes and tell your story. Those who are captivated and intrigued by it will want to know more.

Can Marking Yourself as Disadvantaged Hurt You?

The Disadvantaged Status essay could hurt you if you try to write about something that truly shouldn't be written about. If you've had an experience in your life that you feel is unique to yourself, but when the average person looks at it, they don't think it's unique, you'll likely have some issues. Best case scenario, the reviewer may ignore your essay and not use it as part of their holistic review of your application. The worst-case scenario is they ignore the rest of your application and move on to the next student.

If you are going to write about being disadvantaged, make sure you run it by your advisor, mentor, or another trusted person to see if what you want to talk about is going to be received well. They are not there to tell you *if* you should mark yourself as disadvantaged, but they can tell you how your essay reads.

EXAMPLES

Let's go through some real examples from students.

Race, Ethnicity, and Education

Due to the disparity of primary care physicians, my exposure to Hispanic physicians in the workforce was non-existent. The lack of diversity in the professional healthcare system made me question if my cultural class was equipped for certain societal roles. The lack of minority physicians motivated me. I experienced social disadvantages in the inability to interact with physicians from my social, racial, and educational status. College education was not in my family's cultural norm. The cultural divide prevented me from receiving support others had from their mentors. My community is ranked as one of the least educated towns in California. Only 1% of females within my county obtain a professional degree; a challenge I seek to overcome. As a first-generation college student, I understand racial disparities. I hope to become a role model for other Hispanic women considering medicine. I was told because of my race, I would not be a competitive candidate for medicine; to consider a different career because women were less inclined to complete STEM degrees. I strive to transcend cultural and social biases for the next generation of physicians. Four generations later, I have begun a path that my family has never ventured: to seek a degree in medicine. (1265 characters)

> *This Disadvantaged Status essay does a good job of explaining where the student comes from and the impact on that area on their educational journey. I like the use of numbers, including the "1% of females" statement and how the community is ranked very low in education. The first four sentences seem to repeat the same overall theme that could have likely been said in one sentence: "Growing up interested in medicine, I doubted my abilities, and the abilities of others like me because I never saw a female, Hispanic physician."*
>
> *After that discussion, the student makes a big switch from ethnicity to education, which is also a very important part of being disadvantaged. I don't think the link between first-generation and racial disparities is a good correlation. There are still a lot of White first-generation college students. Unlike the personal statement, I think there is a little room for negativity in the Disadvantaged Status essay to help the reader understand the full scope of your situation.*

Immigrant Parents and First-Generation College Student

As the daughter of immigrants, the sacrifice my parents made moving to an unfamiliar country was never lost on me. I was taught that nothing would be handed to me. I recognized the dedication they maintained in a foreign land to ensure that my sister and I had the opportunities they didn't. But the situation presented itself as a double-edged sword when I discovered that lack of resources and information had been the most significant hurdle to overcome, not only as an applicant but as a senior in high school ignorant of the steps I had to take to enter college. I've been many firsts in my family; a first-generation American, a first-generation high school graduate, now a first-generation college graduate with the last among my proudest accomplishments. I can't say it's been easy. From my parents, I've learned that hard work and persistence are essential to achieving my goals, despite my circumstances. This realization didn't come until entering college where I saw the discrepancies in how I grew up compared to others. While I held a job in school, many of my peers focused on their courses. When my interests shifted to medicine, I struggled to find opportunities to expand my clinical exposure. But my background has taught me that overcoming these hurdles are essential milestones to achieving my dreams. (1322 characters)

This is a good example of an essay that might give me some pause. On the surface, I can imagine how hard it is for a student to navigate the process to college without help from their parents. Looking at data, it looks like one of the biggest disadvantages for first-generation students is finances. Knowledge is everywhere. A web search, YouTube video, or going to an advisor can answer your questions. With the internet, everything you need is a web search away.

The second part of the essay definitely impacts me. As a high school student, needing to contribute to the household income can be a huge detriment to one's ability to take advantage of social and educational opportunities to grow and adapt like your peers. I would focus on that more.

The biggest takeaway I want you to have from this is that a reviewer reading that you are marking yourself as disadvantaged only because you are a first-generation college student may not be received well. Cultural, socioeconomic, and other factors that play into your path as a first-generation college student are what will help the reviewer understand your story more.

I added this paragraph specifically in this book because I have read so many disadvantaged essays that only focus on being a first-generation college student. Those essays do not resonate or tell a story.

> *It is very similar to writing that you want to be a doctor because you want to help people. There needs to be more to the story.*

Immigrant

When I was three, my family immigrated from a life of rummaging for change to buy food in Mexico, to stability in a two-story home in California. However, stability only lasted a few years. My dad was laid off from his job due to his immigration status, forcing my family of five to move into the living room of a single-room duplex. My uncle and his family were kind in offering us to stay under their already crowded roof, but it was difficult for my sisters and I, as we had to use a bucket as a restroom in the middle of the night. We moved to Mexico soon after, and despite our financial hardships and the tension they caused between my parents, my life in Mexico was beautiful. I loved growing up in my grandmother's home and learning more about my culture, but our rural town could not offer the education I sought, so I returned to the US on my own when I was sixteen. I worked at Taco-Bell during my senior year of high school and the first year of junior college, but had to pause my education after receiving an out-of-state tuition bill. In the following years at my junior college and at UC San Diego, I have always had at least one part-time job either in retail, housekeeping, administration, or research. Reflecting on my "disadvantaged" childhood, I have my parents to thank for never feeling that way. (1319 characters)

> *This is a good example of how being an immigrant can turn your world upside down. From being in the country, living in a house, to being forced to use a bucket as a toilet, and going back to Mexico, this student shows their journey. They also throw in some positivity in the end by thanking their parents. This also helps explain a potential red flag in the application, a hiatus in their education. This is well done.*

Undocumented Immigrant

To identify myself as being "a disadvantaged applicant" is both uncomfortable and challenging. It is uncomfortable because it requires comparing myself to what I consider to be the standard medical school applicant. The challenge is figuring out what scale to measure on. What I consider to have been periods of time growing up where I felt disadvantaged, others from starkly different backgrounds may consider privileges. That being said, here are five truths about my upbringing:

1. I spent an extended period of time as an undocumented immigrant with a mother that worked scrubbing floors and an absent father.

2. I qualified for free lunch for the entirety of my time in the public school system.

3. I was the first person in my extended family to gain acceptance into a four-year University.

4. I am the only student in my D-rated public school's recent known history to attend Vanderbilt University.

5. Vanderbilt provided 100% of my financial need but failed to meet the indeterminate needs of a first-generation Latinx student attending an elite university built on the backs of black and brown labor.

I believe that the presentation of these truths will allow the designated medical schools to classify me as either an advantaged or a disadvantaged applicant relative to the rest of the applicant pool. (1312 characters)

> *This is an interesting essay. It does a good job of showing the reviewer what the student has gone through. I don't like the closing paragraph about allowing the medical schools to classify them as either advantaged or disadvantaged. When I think about it, it sounds like the student is turning the Disadvantaged Status essay into a strength, which it's not meant to be. It's not meant to be a sob story either. It's just meant to show why you think you're disadvantaged. The style of "talking to" the reviewer is not something I recommend either. The part about Vanderbilt being built on the backs of black and brown labor also adds a narrative that isn't needed in this specific essay. A better closing would have made this better.*

Immigrant, Caretaker

Five years ago, I moved to the United States for college with my younger sister from China. Moving to a new country was very exciting, especially as I was beginning college, but also very terrifying. However, since it was only my sister and me, I had to set an example for her and take care of her from the dangers of the world and not show her how terrified I was. Integrating into a new culture came with its own difficulties, including learning English as a second language, and homesickness. The addition of me taking care of my sister made it a whole lot more difficult. During our first few months in the US, we had to live in a motel for three months as we did not have a credit history and were two immigrant teenagers who no one wanted to rent to. Sleeping on the motel room couch, going to school and taking my sister to school are not my best memories. One funny example of my newness to the US was that, whenever I drove, I would see the word XING on the ground, and I had no idea what it was. One day I asked my friends who XING was, and they laughed for a while, before telling me that it meant crossing. However, none of these obstacles deterred me from my goal. Instead, they showed me that I could tackle any challenges that I face in life.

This is the essay of the student I mentioned earlier. Even with a 3.9+ GPA and 520+ MCAT, based on this student's story, I would mark as disadvantaged. Your stats don't determine your disadvantaged status—your story does. He does a great job of showing the different aspects of being an immigrant and caretaker. He also throws in a good anecdote about seeing XING on the ground. Any place that you can fit anecdotes into your application, I would tell you to go for it. Well-told stories help your application be more memorable.

ARRESTS, CONVICTIONS, AND INSTITUTIONAL ACTIONS

Having any sort of arrest, conviction, or institutional action on your record can be a sign of poor character or judgment. Having these on your record is not an automatic disqualification from medical school. Yes, medical schools can easily filter out any students who mark yes to these questions, but many times, they'll want to read what happened, and more importantly, what you learned from the experience.

If you have any questions about these prompts and if you need to answer yes to any of these questions, I highly recommend seeking legal counsel.

As with most things, when it comes to these prompts, the details are all in the language used. "Have you ever been arrested?" is a different question than "Have you ever been convicted?" What happens if your conviction was expunged? What if your institutional action doesn't seem to show up on your transcript?

I have recorded two episodes of *The Premed Years* with Larry Cohen, a lawyer who does a lot of medical licensing work. We talked a lot about this topic. You can listen to those episodes at premedyears.com/197 and premedyears.com/399.

As always, you need to fully read the application-specific instruction manual as well. There is a lot of state-specific information that can affect how you will answer these questions.

When you answer yes to any of these questions, each of the application services will open up an additional dialog box for you to enter in your explanation.

TMDSAS gives you 600 characters and asks you to "Explain fully, including dates."

AACOMAS allots 500 characters and asks you to "Include: 1) A brief description of the incident and/or arrest, 2) Specific charge made, 3) Related dates, 4) Consequence, 5) A reflection on the incident and how the incident has impacted your life."

AMCAS has space for 1325 characters and asks you to "Please briefly explain each instance along with the date(s) of occurrence" for institutional actions and to "Please explain the circumstances of your conviction, including the number of conviction(s), the nature of offense(s) leading to conviction(s), date and location of conviction(s), the sentence(s) imposed, and the type(s) of rehabilitation" for misdemeanors or felonies.

There is a right way and a wrong way to offer an explanation. If you were arrested and blame someone else—that is wrong. If you were caught cheating and blame someone else—that is wrong. It ultimately doesn't matter whose fault it is. As I recently said to one student who was trying to deflect blame, "Who is the Admissions Committee going to believe—an academic institution that says you cheated, or a student?"

I was at a conference talking to a premed advisor and a Dean of Admissions at a medical school. They were discussing the advisor's student who was applying to medical school and struggling to get in because they had a student code of conduct infraction for plagiarism on their record, and they weren't accepting blame. Turning their eyes towards me, the Dean asked if I would want that student in my class. Nope!

Personal Statement

Something a lot of students try to do is write about these issues in their personal statement. Because the application services give you space to discuss in a separate text box, I would focus the discussion there. Remember that the personal statement should focus on why you want to be a physician. Distracting the reader with this information may lessen the impact of your story.

EXAMPLES

Let's go through some real examples from students.

Academic Dismissal

In 2011, my daughter was born a stillbirth. I didn't know what I should do so I returned to work on my bachelors. I kept registering for classes hoping that I could push through and return to my former self. However, my grief would take over and I couldn't attend classes. After many failed semesters and an academic dismissal, I decided to take a break from school. I got a job as an EMT and patient care helped to heal me and reignite my passion. In 2015, I returned to school and have excelled since. (503 characters)

This response is hitting most of the things needed to answer the questions AACOMAS asks. We have a brief description of the incident, dates, and consequences. We also have what the student did to take a break and recharge. What we're missing, which would have been nice to fit in, is some reflection on the mistake. A more simplified version of this, which includes some reflection, could look like this: "Still reeling from the loss of my stillborn daughter in 2011, I kept pushing through with classes, failing most of them due to lack of attendance. I realize now that the better decision would have been to take a break sooner. When I finally did take my break, I became an EMT, which reignited my drive and helped me overcome my grief. Since returning to school in 2015, I have been able to return to my previous academic excellence."

Student Code of Conduct Violation

1) I was falsely accused of cheating on an exam by having a notecard and/ or a cellphone 2) Cheating 3) Spring 2018 4) Suspended for one semester 5) During this time, I learned a lot about myself. This event made me strive more for excellence. I was able to transfer to State University. Ever since, my years of college have improved with better academic grades, publications, and awards. In addition, I got the chance to volunteer at low-income clinics and got hired at University Hospital. (490 characters)

As you can see in this example, the student did a few things wrong here. The first thing you should notice is the listed response. Even though AACOMAS numbers what they what to make sure you touch on in your response, your response shouldn't be a numbered list. It should be a narrative in paragraph form. The second thing that should easily be noticeable is the complete lack of accepting blame. The first words, "I was falsely accused," would immediately cause this student's application to be rejected, even with great stats.

Remember—OWN your mistakes. Reflect on the mistake. Here is how it could have been written to take some ownership and show growth: "With easy access to my phone during a test in the Spring of 2018, I was suspended for one semester for cheating as a code of conduct violation. I knew I shouldn't have had my phone with me, and I regret putting myself in that situation. During my suspension, I reflected on my decision making and vowed to start back up at school with a renewed focus and energy on being the best student possible."

Misdemeanor Conviction

This one is a little longer than normal because it was used in a secondary essay since the offense didn't meet the criteria to mark yes on the primary application.

OWI (Operating While Intoxicated) 1st - Traffic Forfeiture. 1 conviction. Date of violation: 1/1/2015. Sentences: 7 months DOT License revocation,

$985.00 fine, Required Interlock Ignition Device for 12 months, Alcohol Assessment, Group Dynamics Highway Safety Course. Voluntary Rehabilitation: University BASICS (Brief Alcohol Screening and Intervention for College Students)

At a friend's cabin, we went to a bar and I offered for our designated driver to use my vehicle. On our way home my vehicle broke down and we were stranded on the side of the road. I chose to climb into the driver seat to try to figure out what the problem was. While trying to determine what happened a squad car pulled up behind us. The officer ran the plates, saw that it was my family's vehicle and saw me in the driver seat with the keys in the ignition under the influence of alcohol. Since this occurred I voluntarily participated in an alcohol use education course (BASICS) and now volunteer for Peer Health Advocates at Personal Decisions Around Alcohol Use events on campus.

> *Similar to the previous example, this student starts with a list. I would change this into a narrative to make it more readable and easier to connect with. The student then explains what happened in the paragraph after but fails to take full responsibility and reflect on the incident. It reads more like bad luck than anything else, but there still should be something like: "I understand that because I was drinking and under the influence of alcohol, I shouldn't have been anywhere near a position of being able to drive the car."*

Institutional Action

This is the same student as the previous response.

October 2015 -On a weekend night, a few friends and I were outside and we chose to urinate in the grass. We were cited for a residence life underage alcohol conduct violation.

April 2016 -On a weekend night, I chose to consume alcohol in a dorm room with friends when a Resident Assistant found us responsible for a residence life underage alcohol conduct violation.

Following these events, I completed the mandatory alcohol education course for first and second on-campus offenses. Although I participated in these courses, the gravity of my actions did not fully hit me until a third, non-University affiliated event in Summer 2017 mentioned in another section of this application. Since that event, I have volunteered with the Peer Health Advocates on campus at "Personal Decisions Around Alcohol Use" events to share my story, and what I have learned about safe alcohol use, with other undergrad students to help them avoid the mistakes I have made. I voluntarily completed a BASICS Program with our Campus Wellness Coordinator. I have grown much closer to my parents than ever before, I have grown tenfold in my Faith, and have gained a significantly strengthened sense of humility and ownership. I continue to spread my message on campus and offer help to those who may also be trying to learn from similar mistakes. (1324 characters)

> *You can see here that the student again listed the incidences. I would have woven them into a narrative. Did the student have to mention urinating? They may have been able to say something else, maintaining transparency, without the specific details. The student also says, "Although I participated in these courses, the gravity of my actions did not fully hit me until a third, non-University affiliated event…" This would be a red flag for me. The student is admitting that they went through the courses but didn't really learn anything from their behavior. They do finish up with some good reflection.*

Academic Probation

In Fall of 2014, and again in Winter of 2016, I was placed on academic probation at Private University for receiving a semester GPA below 2.0. In Fall of 2016, I again received below a 2.0 and was placed on a one-year academic suspension. I recognize that my poor academic performance rests solely on myself. I have since learned to dedicate myself to academic success and shown my abilities in postbac work. I recognize now that in order to become a doctor, you must prove yourself as a student. (496 characters)

This student had significant struggles as a student, being placed on probation twice, and ultimately suspended for one year. They take ownership but don't really explain why it happened in the first place. I would have liked to see some explanation as to why the student thinks it happened. It's ultimately that answer that helps the Admissions Committee understand that trigger and hopefully be there to support the student in the future if ultimately accepted.

Academic Probation

Academic Probation 12/2015 for unsatisfactory performance during the Fall semester of 2015. The probation was lifted after completing the following semester in good standing, 05/2016. (183 characters)

This response doesn't do enough to explain what happened and what was learned.

Misdemeanor Conviction

I was convicted on February 1st, 2016 for a DUI misdemeanor in Dallas, Texas by the city's Superior Court. I was sentenced to pay court fines, complete a 6 month DUI program, and 3 years of unsupervised probation. My dues have been paid, case has been dismissed, and I am awaiting for expungement. However, I was crestfallen at my irresponsibility. I remember staring endlessly in the mirror for weeks coping, but I realized that the only real setback in life is death. I ceased alcohol consumption, made healthier lifestyle choices, and attended my Church's service to seek forgiveness. I became involved with a community of recovering addicts, and I used the time in my DUI program to hear the stories of substance abuse victims and understand their health-related decisions. I would never advise someone to learn this way, but failure can be used to empower ourselves and others. I told my group to call me whenever they felt a relapse, and talk about ways to use their struggle in a positive manner. It is a high to be able to observe our efforts for others in need. This perspective reinforced my desire to protect those who face adversity. Every experience in my life has taught me some self-improvement. I will have more challenges ahead, but the messages I take along are only going to make me a more fit physician. (1323 characters)

> *This student does a great job of hitting on all of the requested details, owning their mistakes and reflecting on the experience.*

Student Code of Conduct Violation

There is a citation for alcohol use on my conduct record with State University. On 10/31/16, upon returning to the dorm, I was accused of using alcohol. During my subsequent meeting with the dorm manager, I admitted to using alcohol because it was the truth and I needed to take responsibility. I was required to attend a counseling session, write a short essay, and pay a $35 fine. I reflected on my choice that night and my future actions are emblematic of the impact of this as I never had another violation. (511 characters)

> *This response is close to being very good. It hits all the basic information needed, and with a few tweaks, it could be perfect. Saying "I was accused" makes it sound like the student was deflecting blame, yet in the next sentence, they admit to drinking. I think it could have been left out completely. Here is a rewrite that tries to say the same thing with a little deeper reflection: "While still underage on 10/31/16, I had a lapse in judgment and drank alcohol at a party. Later, when it was brought to the attention of my dorm manager, I admitted the mistake, attended a counseling session, wrote a short essay, and paid a $35 fine. Reflecting on the choices I made that night, I realize that my actions were not up to the standards I need to maintain as a future professional, and I keep that thought with me to this day."*

Marijuana

During my Freshman year of college, I desperately wanted to fit into the rest of my freshman class, which I had unsuccessfully accomplished during my high school career. In doing so, this led me to hang out with individuals who were fully immersed in the more social aspects of college. As a result, I received 3 points for the possession of marijuana paraphernalia, which was expunged after avoiding disciplinary action for 3 terms.

This experience forced me to reevaluate my freshman experience and refocus my ultimate goals for college. Subsequently, I decided to focus more on academics and develop friendships with individuals who possessed similar goals to myself. Now 3 years removed from this disciplinary action, I can say that I no longer require the approval of others and I am more confident in myself and my goals. (826 characters)

You can see from this experience that the student did a good job of owning the issue. They struggled with fitting in, fell into the wrong crowd, and made some bad decisions. You immediately see improvement with the discipline being expunged after three terms. And finally, you can see the student reflected on the experience and showed growth by changing their perspective. This is a good example of how to talk about your red flags.

WORK AND ACTIVITIES

The work and activities section, or as many call it, the extracurricular section of the application, is one of the hardest parts of the primary application. You've hopefully done a lot of different things up to this point, and you want to talk about them forever, but you're very limited with the character count the applications give you; additionally, AMCAS limits you with the total number you can add.

If you are a nontraditional student, you may have 30 or 40 potential things to list—how do you choose? If you're a traditional student who has focused on your grades and MCAT score, you may only have five. Is that enough?

Let's first talk about some of the application specifics for extracurriculars.

APPLICATION SPECIFICS

AMCAS

AMCAS gives you a maximum of 15 activities to include. You are allowed up to 700 characters to write a description of each activity.

You can designate up to three activities as most meaningful. Doing so will give you a *separate* 1325 character essay box to write about why it was most meaningful. When you designate an activity as most meaningful, the prompt you are given is:

> *This is your opportunity to summarize why you have selected this experience as one of your most meaningful. In your remarks, you might consider the transformative nature of the experience: the impact you made while engaging in the experience and the personal growth you experienced as a result of your participation.*

Notice how the prompt does not mention anything about medicine. Too many students ignore what are truly meaningful and transformative moments in their life because they think they have to focus on "most meaningful for being a physician." Really dig through your experiences and focus on the most meaningful to you as a person, and not necessarily those related to your journey to medical school.

The categories for the AMCAS activities are:
- Artistic Endeavors
- Community Service/Volunteer - Medical/Clinical
- Community Service/Volunteer - Not Medical Clinical
- Conferences Attended
- Extracurricular Activities
- Hobbies
- Honors/Awards/Recognitions
- Intercollegiate Athletics
- Leadership - Not Listed Elsewhere
- Military Service

- Other
- Paid Employment - Medical/Clinical
- Paid Employment - Not Medical/Clinical
- Physician Shadowing/Clinical Observation
- Presentations/Posters
- Publications
- Research/Lab
- Teaching/Tutoring/Teaching Assistant

For AMCAS, you will need to provide the start date (month and year), end date (month and year), total hours, and contact info for potential verification. For activities like hobbies, or others where there is no contact info, put yourself.

AACOMAS

AACOMAS doesn't have a limit on the number of activities that you can include. You are allowed up to 600 characters to write a description of that activity.

In AACOMAS, there are no designations for most meaningful activities.

The categories for the AACOMAS activities are:

- Non-healthcare Employment
- Extracurricular Activities
- Non-healthcare Volunteer or Community Enrichment
- Healthcare Experience

For AACOMAS activities, you will need to provide the start date, end date (if not still ongoing), average weekly hours, and number of weeks. Contact info is not mandatory, but I would recommend it.

AACOMAS also has a separate section on the application called "Achievements."

The categories for the AACOMAS achievements are:

- Awards
- Honors
- Presentations

- Publications
- Scholarships

For AACOMAS achievements, you need to provide the name, presenting organization, date, and description.

TMDSAS

TMDSAS does things a little differently with activities. They have what is called a "Personal Biography" that lists different activity types and asks you if you have anything for that section. If you mark yes, then you can enter the necessary information. You are allowed up to 300 characters to write a description of that activity. Like AACOMAS, there is no limit to the number of activities you can include.

TMDSAS allows you to designate up to three activities as most meaningful, which gives you a *separate* 500 characters to write about those activities.

The sections of the Personal Biography for TMDSAS are:
- Academic Recognition
- Non-Academic Recognition
- Leadership
- Employment
- Research Activities
- Healthcare Activities
- Veterinary Supervised Experience
- Animal Experience
- Community Service
- Extracurricular & Leisure
- Meaningful Experiences
- Planned Activities

For TMDSAS, you will need to provide the start date (month and year), end date (month and year), and hours worked per week.

How Old Can Activities Be?

There are no hard and fast rules when it comes to how far back you can go for your activities. AACOMAS recommends within the last ten years and "at the collegiate level and above."

The generally accepted practice for all of the application services is that included activities should be after high school. The exception to this is if you have an experience that you started while in high school that you carried over into college and beyond. You can put your start date back as far as you need. You should not, however, include an experience that happened solely in high school, even if it was a meaningful and transformative experience.

Don't confuse this practice for the activities section with your personal statement. The personal statement often will include an experience that happened during or before high school. The experiences you are writing about in your personal statement that show why you want to be a doctor can go back as far as you need.

For nontraditional applicants, some meaningful experiences happened more than ten years ago. I wouldn't discourage you from adding these to your activities list as long as you can show the reader that they were important to you. Use your judgment as to whether or not you want to add something that is older.

Choosing Activities

If you go back to the prior chapter about the core competencies, you will get a good idea of what medical schools may be looking for in an applicant and future medical student. You can use these core competencies to figure out which extracurriculars to include if you need to cut some out.

Ultimately, every time you add a new activity, the questions you should be asking yourself are:

- Why am I including this here?
- Is this experience something I want to write about right now?
- Does it make me excited to think about this experience?
- Will I be enthusiastic to talk about this experience during my interviews?
- Is this something that has impacted me or something that shows my impact?

You should be able to discuss everything that you include in your activities list during your interviews. If you are uncomfortable talking about something on your list, then you probably shouldn't include it. If there was research that you did, but you hated the research, and you did not get along with the principal investigator, then you might not want to put it on the list. If you had a job that didn't mean much to you and was only about a paycheck without really having any impact on you at all, you might not want to put that on your application either.

Ask yourself, "What is this showing the Admissions Committee about me? Is it just showing them that I did something, or is it showing them the type of person I am and the type of impact I will have as part of their next medical school class?"

Not every activity is going to be amazing. A lot of things you add are going to be there to show a timeline of what you have done and aren't necessarily activities that made a huge impact on your life or highlight a core competency. That is okay, too.

Most Meaningful Activities

A common question I get from students is, "Which one of my activities should I mark as most meaningful?" Or, "Are the activities I have selected as most meaningful unique, or should I choose other activities?"

Asking someone else what activities are the most meaningful to *you* doesn't make sense, does it? I know where the students are coming from—they are trying to figure out which of their activities *best* highlight who they are to get the attention of the Admissions Committees. They are trying to "stand out."

The truth is that you should not try to "figure out" what the Admissions Committee is looking for; rather, you should focus on your story, your strengths, and your passions. Pick the activities that are truly the most meaningful to *you*, which is all the Admissions Committee wants to see.

If being a soccer coach was a meaningful experience for *you*, put that in your application. If you've traveled extensively, and those are meaningful experiences for you, then they can be the most meaningful experiences in your application. This is your story. Own your story and help others see it as well.

How to Combine Activities

For the AMCAS application, which limits you to 15 activities, there are some opportunities to combine many different activities into one activity spot to save space.

Shadowing is usually one of the easiest to combine, as it is typically a passive experience, and individual shadowing experiences don't need to be highlighted in a description. There may be exceptions to this that you want to highlight in a separate spot, but for most students, you can combine all of your shadowing into one activity and add just one contact information. You can combine all the hours and dates and add those to the activity details. In your description, you can list the different physicians you shadowed and put a very brief timeline in there as well. Fit what you can and know that it doesn't have to include everything—it just needs to show that you've been busy shadowing.

Honors/Awards/Recognitions and presentations are also very easy to combine into one activity. Unless there is a specific activity you want to keep separate, I would combine as much as you can into one activity.

Combining Multiple Positions at the Same Location

It is very common for you to have held multiple positions at the same location. If you're a military vet, you will have had many roles while in the military. Does that mean you should enter all of them? If you started at a premed club as a general member during your Freshman year and were elected president your Senior year, how do you combine those?

For AMCAS, you will have to be careful with how much you separate roles because of the 15 activity limit. For AACOMAS and TMDSAS, there is much less concern, and you can do what you want.

I generally don't recommend breaking things out into more than two activities. In your AMCAS application, if you're a military vet, you may want to use one activity to highlight the core of your role in the military and the other activity to highlight a leadership position. It's the same for the student who was part of the premed club. Highlight your role as a member and the impact you had as a member, and then use another activity to write about your impact as an officer of the club.

How to Write the Activity Description

Before I delve into how to write the activity description, let me show you an email I received recently from a student. While I never interacted with this student directly, they took my advice in my YouTube videos to craft their application.

> *Today, I had an interview with UF College of Medicine (Go Gators!) and I had the most incredible time speaking with faculty and students about my journey towards medicine. In every interaction I had with faculty and students who reviewed my file, they remembered me and praised the way I told stories in my experience/ extracurricular section of my AMCAS. I really want to thank you for the time and resources you provided me in how to write for the experience section of AMCAS, as well as my personal statement. Your personal statement book was PHENOMENAL, and I have recommended it to so many friends and loved ones applying. It wholeheartedly is the reason I believe schools like UF wanted to get to know me and extended an interview invite."*

They emailed me a few days later after receiving an acceptance!

Like we talked about in the personal statement chapter, your story and how you are able to capture it can be very impactful.

We talked earlier about how many characters you have for each description. The AMCAS application only allows 700 characters. TMDSAS and AACOMAS give you even less. As I've said, I believe that writing the description of the activities is harder than writing the personal statement. Considering there is less space yet so much to say, students struggle to do this well.

Where most students go wrong with the activity description is that they write a generic job description that I could easily copy and paste into another student's application. If you are writing your activity descriptions generically, and you are not showing who *you* are but rather what the position was, then you need to go back to the drawing board.

Here is an example of an activity description that I could easily copy and paste into someone else's application and one that doesn't show me who the student is or their impact. This student also starts to dive into "selling," which we'll talk about as well.

> *This family medicine clinic sees thousands of patients, from infants to the elderly, on a daily basis. As a scribe and medical assistant, I was trained on the job to assist with improving general office workflow and management of charts and electronic documentation. Through my role, I was able to shorten wait times, increase patient satisfaction, and assist in minor in-office medical procedures such as cleaning wounds and taking vitals. (440 characters)*

Here's another example of some generic information about being a TA.

> *I was recommended by my professor to serve as a TA. I created lesson plans and learned how to command attention from my students. I became skilled in teaching broad concepts of chemistry. I gave my students the space to explore and challenged them to think deeper about how to learn chemistry. I learned how to adjust the intensity of our discussions to their level of understanding and education. All of my students are on a different level, and some experience more difficulties. (481 characters)*

You may read this and think it's great—the student did a good job telling the reader how they were able to challenge the students and adjust to their needs. When I read this, I say, "Yes, that is what a TA (or any teacher/professor) does." There is nothing specific here that shows me who this student is. What would have made it stronger is a story of the applicant working with one individual student—a situation that can't be replicated by any other student.

Here is an example of a student telling a story of interacting with a student as a TA.

> *The first time I held office hours as a teaching assistant, 3 chemistry PhD candidates were the sole attendees. I started by fielding questions regarding lecture material. As we turned our attention to the homework, they expressed frustration that the assignment did not align with what had been taught in*

class. I went through the prompt and rephrased the question. There was a collective "oh" from the students and they began to frantically write responses. Each week the same three students returned and each week they performed exceptionally well. Over time, they learned to use the strategies I taught them to detect the nuances in the questions and rely on my explanations less and less.

This is a specific story of working with PhD students and helping them figure out their homework. It could have been stronger if it was one-on-one, but I think it is better than the previous example.

What is Your Impact?

Try to write your extracurricular descriptions in a way that highlights you. What was the impact that you had on the position? What was an experience you can write about that impacted you? For instance, if you volunteered at hospice, don't just say you were given assignments and you spent time with patients at their houses reading to them or holding their hands until they passed. Everyone at hospice does that.

Tell the story of one patient. Describe an interaction with them. Describe how it made you feel and how your presence made them feel. Write about that impact, because you are the only one who had that very specific experience with that one patient. That is what makes for a good activity description.

Here's an example of a student's experience working as an interventional radiology tech.

"Mrs. Hoban" grabbed onto my hand as I placed the ECG leads on her frail body lying on the procedure table. I looked into her eyes and saw confusion, terror, and anxiety. With ample staff present to set up for surgery I decided to hold her hand as I spoke to her calmly and quietly to reduce the fear within her. She was having a stroke. Once Mrs. Hoban was intubated, I scrubbed into the thrombectomy procedure to assist as the physicians attempted to remove the cerebral clot from her brain. The privilege of learning interventional neurology has been a pinnacle experience. Working

in interventional radiology, interventional cardiology and electrophysiology have been challenging and rewarding. (699 characters)

Instead of *telling* the reader about his empathy, teamwork, and ability to handle a stressful situation, this student *showed* the reader these qualities through a story, without selling himself. This student was able to do all of that in less than 700 characters.

Just like the personal statement, the goal is to *show*, not *tell*. Unfortunately, the TMDSAS application doesn't give you enough room to do that with only 300 characters. There is room to do it well in your AMCAS and AACOMAS applications, however. I'll have some more examples at the end of this chapter.

Where is the "So What?"

My co-host on Ask the Dean and our VP of Academic Advising at Mappd, Dr. Scott Wright, loves to use the phrase "It's not about the what, it's about the so what." I love this phrase because it concisely focuses on what I just spent many words saying. The *what* is the basic job description that students love to write about. The *so what* is the impact you realize through reflection.

Non-medical Activities

If you are writing about something non-medical, you can add numbers to show your impact. If you were on a sales team, how much money did you add to the team? If you were in charge of philanthropy in a sorority, how much money did you raise, or how many volunteer projects did you organize? Showing your impact through money raised or lives impacted is a great way to show who you are, instead of just saying you organized events for the sorority sisters.

Here is a good example of what that may look like.

I joined the LGBT Health Workforce Conference as a Social Media Director, where I worked closely with the planning committee to develop our first Facebook outreach initiative. By designing engaging visuals and social media posts, we drove targeted engagement, and contributed to increasing both the number of registrants and abstracts submitted. Our 2017 conference registered more than 300 health professionals, and received over 60 abstracts, a 10% and 50% increase from 2016, respectively. I learned that empowering our healthcare professionals to better address the needs of LGBT individuals is a crucial step towards lessening health disparities that disproportionately impact this community. (697 characters)

This student does a great job showing the reader the impact through numbers—300 health professionals and 60 abstracts—and the increase in those numbers. Although the conference was geared towards healthcare, the activity itself isn't, yet it still shows the student's impact.

Here are some other things to think about to show impact for a non-clinical activity like being a salesperson:

- Did you run a campaign for a company as a salesperson?
- How much money did you make the company?
- Did you win any awards as a salesperson?
- Were you the top salesperson in your company?
- Did you streamline any processes to improve sales at your company?

Highlight very specific facts. If you ran a donation drive as part of a premed club as an undergrad, talk specifically about how much money was raised, how many clothes were donated, how much food was contributed. Talk specifics to show the impact. If you were the president of your premed club, don't just talk about organizing premed meetings and organizing recruitment for the club. Talk specifically about how many speakers you brought in, how many members you led, how much money was being raised and budgeted and managed under your watch as president. When you are able to show specific numbers, it shows the impact you were able to have on the position.

Write in Paragraphs

With the possible exception of the combined activities we've already talked about, when you are writing your descriptions, do not bullet point your description lists. Write in full sentences and avoid writing as you would on a résumé. Sentences that start with "Taught," "Ensured," "Led," "Made," or

"Encouraged" are all very common ways to write a résumé. Don't do this for your descriptions.

Don't Waste Characters

With so little room in your descriptions, do not make the common mistake of adding wasted characters. Every activity, outside of the description, includes the details about how many hours you spent, the name of the organization, and where it took place. Many students like to repeat some of these details in their description.

Examples:

- I joined Theta Chi Fraternity during my sophomore year.
- I worked x# of hours per week/month.
- I volunteered every Friday.
- I have been working on this project for 40-50 hours a week since August 2018.
- I shadowed Dr. Smith at University Hospital for 3 months.

Use All of Your Characters

The application is your chance to tell your story. If you are continuously leaving a lot of empty space in your activity descriptions, you are losing out on opportunities to tell that story.

For students applying to both AMCAS and AACOMAS, I recommend writing the description for AMCAS first and then cutting out 100 characters to make it fit the 600 character count for AACOMAS, rather than using the same 600 character count descriptions for both AMCAS and AACOMAS. This is harder and will take more time, but it will give you the ability to flush out your stories for AMCAS.

Examples

This first example is a good representation of the applicant showing the reader what it was like being a server.

One of my favorite tasks as a server at Winery was to give tours of the facility. Every weekend people from all over the country would come to sample our locally produced wine, and I would guide them through the basics of how they were made. I especially enjoyed walking the group through the cellar that held our oak barrels. Some were undergoing malolactic fermentation, causing a gentle bubbling of CO2 to escape from the airlocks. Many others were quietly aging reds that had been placed there several months up to a few years before, and a few were from grapes I had helped to harvest. From vine to glass, it was rewarding to be an integral part of the winemaking process. (677 characters)

This is how many students would write about the activity:

Provided wine samples to customers. Gave tours to customers. Harvested grapes for winemaking. Improved communication skills by talking to customers from all over the country. Made sure that every customer was taken care of. Worked as an integral member of the team to ensure the winemaking process went smoothly.

You can see that in the first example, there is a lot of *showing*—I can visualize the oak barrels, smell the fermentation, and hear the CO2 escaping. The student wasn't trying to *sell* anything to the reader. As the reader, I can tell the student interacted a lot with people, so the student probably has good communication skills. It is evident in the writing that the student was a part of the process, meaning they probably are a good team player. I can extrapolate a lot about the student without the student needing to *sell* me on their skills.

In the second example, you can see that the writing is like a résumé, and the student is trying to *sell* me on their specific skills. None of what is written is specific to the student—it is more generic to the position.

Here is another student's actual description of being a server; you decide how you would rate it—closer to the good example or closer to the bad example.

I have worked in a restaurant setting for most of my college career and it has prepared me like no other experience to handle the workload of college. As a waitress I learned the ability to multitask and focus in many environments. It was during this time of employment that I also understood the purpose and importance of building guest relations. (348 characters)

I hope you can see that this description is closer to the bad example. The student is trying to *sell* the skills they learned as a server. It is also only 348 characters and submitted in the AMCAS application. The student left a lot of empty space and failed to show their impact on the position.

In this next example, ask yourself if this student tried to *sell* you on anything. Ask yourself if the description is a generic job description or if it's a story that is specific to the student. This example is one of being a tutor, which is a common premed activity.

My first semester of tutoring, I was paired with "Charlie," a 45-year-old physics major and veteran. Charlie cared more about learning the information than his grade. He was motivated to do well on every assignment, lab, and test, and always seemed fully focused. One day, near the end of the semester, Charlie sat down and said with a smile, "I changed my major to chemistry!" I was stunned, and thrilled. I had made an impact on Charlie's life and had been a part of his discovery of his love for chemistry. This fueled my motivation to build a career in higher education. (574 characters)

Here is how many students would write about the activity:

Tutored students in chemistry. Created lesson plans for students and checked in on their progress. Listening to their specific situations, I was able to craft lessons to the needs of each student. Met with students weekly to answer all of their questions. Helped students prepare for tests.

Again, you can see in the good example above that the student is giving a specific example of an experience as a tutor. Everyone knows what a tutor does. You don't need to list exactly what you were doing—focus on you and your impact, the *so what*. You can see the good example is also less than 600 characters, so it will easily work for AACOMAS, and there is a little room to add to the story for AMCAS.

In the bad example, you can again read a list of basic job tasks that do not help the Admissions Committee see who you are.

Here is a real example from a student talking about tutoring. Where do you think it lands?

As a tutor for physics and chemistry, I took bulky concepts and broke them down into manageable parts for my students to digest. The thrill of helping a student master a concept that had previously stumped them sparked my passion for teaching others. Acquiring the ability to teach to different learning styles not only benefited my students; it helped me realize that everyone learns information at their own pace and in their own way. I believe that mastering the art of simple, effective teaching and guidance will help me to better connect with my patients as I explain complex diagnoses and treatment plans. (612 characters)

This example is a very common one. Students will take what they have done in their experience and then *sell* to the reader why it will help them as a physician. Your job is not to draw these comparisons. You are not a physician. You don't personally know what it will be like to be a physician. Show your impact without selling how it is going to help you in the future as a physician.

I'll have a lot more examples at the end of the chapter.

Should I Include Hobbies?

One of the most common questions I get about the activities section is whether or not to include hobbies. Remember that the activities section isn't to only highlight healthcare-related activities; it is your chance to show who you are as a person through everything you have done, or are currently doing.

I've seen students write about amazing hobbies in their applications. They have done so in a way that highlights who they are as an individual and what their interests are outside of becoming a physician and being a student. For AMCAS, be aware that if you have over 15 activities, your hobbies could bump out another activity. You can avoid this by combining multiple hobbies into one activity to highlight a few different interests you have.

Remember, the goal of the whole application process, after you have shown you are academically capable, is to get a medical school to be interested in you, invite you for an interview, and ultimately accept you. Hobbies are a great way for medical schools to connect with you and understand who you are.

Here's an example of a good hobby description.

I was fourteen when I discovered tap dancing was one of my passions. Although I joined our local dance center because of my initial interest in hip-hop, tap dancing quickly captivated me. After seeing a tap show, I registered for classes, and was soon infatuated with this dance style. I found myself practicing anywhere and everywhere I could. With persistence, I quickly mastered the basics, and I became one of the youngest to join the local center's advanced tap ensemble. Because dancing was perceived as a women's activity, I had to fight against the prejudice of many male friends and family members since a young age. Dancing has taught me to be confident, determined, and true to myself.

What is the Minimum Number of Activities I Should Have?

I mentioned earlier that AMCAS gives you up to 15 slots. AACOMAS and TMDSAS give you an unlimited number of activities to fill in. If you're like many students and only have eight or nine solid activities, you may be worried and think, "I need to go do more things, so I have fifteen."

In truth, you do not need to fill in every activity in the application. It is very easy for an Admissions Committee member to read an application and see which activities were thrown in at the last minute to fluff up the application. The biggest takeaway I want you to have is that **quality** activities always win over the **quantity** of activities.

My recommendation is to have at least ten impactful activities to write about for your application. Some of you may not have ten, and that's just something you will have to navigate when you apply. I wouldn't delay an application only to add more activities to your list unless it is because you don't have recent, consistent clinical experience or shadowing.

What if I Have Fewer Activities Because I'm a Parent/Nontraditional Premed?

As a nontraditional applicant with less time to do activities, when you are filling out your activity list and looking only at what other students are writing about, you may feel like what you have done is not enough.

Medical schools can see everything you are putting on your application; thus, they can see if you work full-time or if you are in school full-time, and they understand you are not going to have the same profile as a 22-year-old traditional student who doesn't have any other responsibilities outside of school. Don't worry about those comparisons because they are truly apples to oranges, and schools know that and can account for it.

Can I Update Activities?

After you submit your applications, there are very minimal edits you can make. If you received a promotion at your job, you will not be able to add that to an existing experience. In AACOMAS, you can add new experiences after you submit your application, but you can't edit old ones.

EXAMPLES

The examples that follow are real examples from students. For some of them, I have before and after feedback that I gave to students. For all of them, I've provided some commentary to help you understand what is good and what could be improved. None of the examples have been edited for grammar or punctuation.

Research

I performed research for a summer internship at the Neuroradiology Laboratory of Dr. Smith. I worked both on the clinical and animal research side focusing on the study of cerebral saccular aneurysms. My responsibilities included chart review looking at the accuracy of ICD9 codes, which helped advance my skills in the research software. I had the opportunity to see both the clinical application of using microcoils to treat aneurysms and be a part of the lab animal research to better understand the mechanisms of aneurysm growth and healing. I was required to learn a large, diverse set of skills in a short amount of time, which strengthened my time management skills. (673 characters)

> *I would consider the first sentence of this activity description to be wasted characters. This information will be in the details that you provide with your description. The student is also combining several common mistakes, including listing their job responsibilities and selling their skills—"helped advance my skills" and "strengthened my time management skills." Most of what is written could be copied to another student's application without any issue.*

Here is the next draft:

As a research student at the Neuroradiology Laboratory of Dr. Smith, I worked both on the clinical and animal research side focusing on the study of cerebral saccular aneurysms. I will never forget my first day walking up to our animal research lab, as I opened the door a sign said "Caution: Pigs at Play." This made me chuckle, but at the same time scared me because I realized just how little I knew about the broad application of animal testing. I had the opportunity to see both the clinical application of using microcoils to treat aneurysms and be a part of the lab animal research to better understand the mechanisms of aneurysm growth and healing. (657 characters)

> *You can see here that we are given a personal story that highlights the student. "Caution: Pigs at Play" is a great visual. We're given a little insight into the student's personality with the chuckle and being*

> *scared. The student didn't try to sell us on their time management or software skills. This is a much better description. The first sentence still has some wasted characters, but the student felt like it helped give a little context to start the story.*

Research

Research was always one of the domains I wanted to explore. I volunteered in research about sleep apnea twice a week, where I analyzed and arranged data using Ponemah and Excel. Then, I was offered a job by the supervisor to work in the lab as a student assistant. I was thrilled to accept this position alongside my other job as a medical scribe. My work primarily focuses on reporting on results and helping with manuscript data for publication. So far, I have learned how to generate, read, and analyze data and how to troubleshoot problems. Additionally, my teamwork skills have improved significantly and I learned how good collaboration with other team members produces the best results. (693 characters)

> *This example highlights what so many students do with their activity descriptions. This tells me nothing about the student and is only used to highlight the job description and sell teamwork and collaboration. Remember that the goal of these descriptions is to show who YOU are, not just want you did and what you think you gained from it.*

Most Meaningful for the above example:

Being involved in this research about sleep apnea has increased my knowledge about sleep stages and the various issues associated with sleep dramatically. Whenever I encounter a new concept, I almost immediately begin researching supporting literature so I can widen my understanding. I have enjoyed the scientific environment in the lab as I work side-by-side with a microbiologist and having the chance to directly observe scientific concepts that I have only seen demonstrated in textbooks up to this point in my education. During the weekly meetings we have with the supervisor, I present my findings and results. I also have the opportunity to ask questions to further my knowledge and clarify any sources of confusion. As a fast learner and multitasker, I was able to contain the huge amount of data that were generated weekly which helped in progressing the manuscript fast; that has just been published in AJRCCM journal for peer reviews. This experience has shown me medicine from a different perspective and has developed in me a sense of reliability. As I continue to work in the lab, I am exploring the realm of scholarly research and continuing to grow my interest in medical research. I plan to continue working in this fascinating line of work for the next several months. (1287 characters)

Remember that the goal of the most meaningful designation is to talk about, ideally through a story, why the experience has been the most meaningful to you as a person. Instead, this student used the most meaningful essay as an opportunity to continue the description with more about what they did and to sell other aspects of their skills and traits.

Research

Patients with retinitis pigmentosa have a mutation in a subdomain of an enzyme called Inosine-5'-Monophosphate Dehydrogenase (IMPDH). While scientists know that this mutation exists, they are unsure how it contributes to the disease process. Using E.coli as a model organism I used the funding from the Fellows Program to better understand the subdomain of IMPDH. The goal was to identify proteins or other macromolecules that interacted with the enzyme so we could better characterize the protein's non-enzymatic functions. Ultimately, we hope to use my findings to better characterize human IMPDH and possibly identify a way to treat a debilitating disease. (659 characters)

While this research description does not tell a story, it educates without trying to sell the reader on the skills gained from doing the research. It doesn't specifically say in this description, but one could assume the student helped get the funding from the Fellows Program, which is a great accomplishment, too.

Customer Service

Beginning in 2014 I was given the opportunity to work as a server at an upscale restaurant in town. It was my responsibility to make sure that orders were taken, entered correctly and delivered to our patrons in a timely manner. Another advantage was the proximity to the hospital which granted me the opportunity to hear about unique patient experiences with my clientele outside of just simple dining. Being a server allowed me to further enhance my customer service skills and abilities to interact with a large breadth of diverse people and unique needs. It has also taught me valuable time management skills of juggling the demands of school and work. (656 characters)

> *How many of you don't know that a server's job is to take orders, enter them correctly, and deliver the food? Job descriptions aren't needed for almost everything that you are going to be adding to your activities list. If there is a random activity that you think needs some explanation, go ahead, but keep it brief. This student is also selling their customer service skills as well as their ability to interact with a diverse set of people. Being a server requires that you have at least some baseline level of customer service and communication skills. You don't need to sell those things.*

Most meaningful for the above example:

For some, waiting tables wouldn't be a job they would be proud of, but for me it has been one of my most rewarding experiences. It has taught me how to thrive under pressure. You have to be able to take care of several tables, each with their own unique needs from a kid spilling their milk, to someone on a low salt diet. It reminds me of the demands of a physician where they might see 15-20 patients in one day all with individual illnesses. Similar to a physician, it was always important for me to remain calm with each guest, no matter how crazy things were.

Waitressing has taught me the art of customer service. It is often the little details that customers remember, rather than the meal itself. "Personalization" is what comes to mind when I think of my service. I have learned that it is not only paying attention to each individual preference, but remembering their needs on their next visit. This is similar to a physician's dictation of clinical notes. With our restaurant's close proximity to the hospital, my guests dine regularly during their follow up visits. One of my guests Phil liked to come to my restaurant every Sunday. He enjoyed a specific booth with a pillow for his back. When I saw his name on the reservation list, I made sure his booth was reserved with a pillow. (1296 characters)

> *You can see the student is really pushing hard to sell why being a server was most meaningful, not really to them, but for their future as a physician. I don't recommend trying to compare anything in your application to medicine. The student claims that working as a server has the same demands as those of a physician. Any physician would probably laugh at the naivety of that comment. I can understand why the student was trying to make that connection, but it comes off poorly.*
>
> *In the second paragraph, you can see more ties to medicine with physicians dictating notes. However, I'm not really sure I understand the connection that is trying to be made between dictating and individual preference. The story told at the end is the best part of this description, and where I want you to focus for your whole description or most meaningful essays. Picture the student getting a pillow ready for the guest—this* shows *the reader their customer service skills. It* shows *the reader that they care and will go above and beyond. This is how you should write your descriptions.*

Here is the next draft:

Waitressing has taught me the art of customer service as its the small details customers remember, rather than the meal itself. "Personalization" is what comes to mind when I think of my service. It is not only paying attention to each individual preference, but remembering their needs on their next visit. One of my guests, Phil, liked to come to my restaurant every Sunday. He enjoyed a specific booth with a pillow for his back. When I saw his name on the reservation list, I made sure his booth was reserved with a pillow. After many visits, Phil wrote on his receipt "Many thanks for always making me feel special, I look forward to our conversations every week." (669 characters)

> *You can see that the student held on to some of the themes they really wanted to focus on. I'm not sure I would have kept them, but they were important to them. They jump into the story of Phil here, which is great.*

Most meaningful for the above example:

The restaurants close proximity to the hospital granted me the opportunity to hear about unique patient experiences with my clientele outside of simple dining. I still vividly remember a couple come in, wife pushing her husband in a wheelchair. When I got to their table, they had papers spread all over and appeared very distressed, their faces blank. The wife explained to me that they went for a second opinion, and received a very difficult and different diagnosis than they had received back home. I could tell they really just needed someone to listen to their concerns. I had a couple other tables at the time, but felt this table needed my attention. My co-workers took on my other tables allowing me to sit down with this struggling couple. I listened as his wife tearfully explained that her husband had been seeking treatment for over a year for a condition he didn't even have. They both were in denial, and heartbroken about his new diagnoses which meant moving their lives to seek treatment. (1005 characters)

> *With this draft, instead of focusing on selling specific skills or traits, the student went right into another story to highlight experiences. They talk about recognizing that this couple needed someone to listen to without saying, "I used my outstanding listening skills to provide them with what they needed." This most meaningful essay is great but could have been made even a little better with a quick reflection on why it was meaningful.*

Shadowing

I was very eager to know more deeply about clinical life, which drove me to shadow an Endocrinologist. Endocrinology was always my interest due to the fact that my brother has a pituitary tumor. I had the opportunity to watch the patients closely, hear their complaints and feel their worries. Throughout days, I developed more compassion and relatedness to the patients. I also got to know a wide range of diagnoses that I had not known before. The knowledge that I developed during my shadowing, and my passionate and enthusiastic made me able to go further and to volunteer as a scribe in the clinic. (603 characters)

> *For most students, shadowing is not very engaging. The majority of the time, you're watching what is going on without much interaction. Writing about these experiences can be very hard, and I usually recommend students just list their shadowing experience(s). Application reviewers understand what shadowing is and are not expecting the world from you. This description is okay for what it is and actually gives a little insight into the student's life with the mention of their brother's pituitary tumor.*

Shadowing

The following three shadowing examples are from the same student, on the same application.

Shadowing Dr. Smith allowed me to see more of the surgical side of being a physician. I was able to observe surgical procedures that include a skin cancer removal from the hand, an abdominoplasty, breast reconstruction, and breast reduction. He also informed me with in depth knowledge of the business side of a private practice and insurance companies. (353 characters)

Shadowing Dr. White provided me with a great opportunity to see the clinical and surgical side of being a physician. Much of his clinical work deals with seeing patients that deal with Gastroesophageal Reflux Disease, throat cancers, hearing aids, and ear infections which are more commonly seen in young children. I was able to see a range of patients from six months old to eighty years old, as well as his different approach to properly caring for each of them. I was also given the opportunity to observe and take part in different procedures surgical and nonsurgical, such as a laryngoscopy, removal of tonsils, and a thyroid removal. (639 characters)

In my time shadowing Dr. Jones, I was able to observe clinical consultations and care, but also able to participate in them. Dr. Jones allowed me the opportunity to talk to certain patients about symptoms they were experiencing and ask them what he called "interview questions" as part of his diagnostic process. This experience allowed me to compare the differences in patient care from family practitioners to other specialty physicians. (439 characters)

You can see from these three descriptions that they are all very basic and generic examples of a student shadowing a physician with no big breakthroughs in how the student was impacted. I don't expect that from shadowing, and neither does the Admissions Committee. Because this student used three separate activities to include shadowing, it looks more like the student is trying to "fluff" up their application due to a lack of activities. These three separate activities could have easily been included in one activity with a bulleted list of the different specialties and physicians shadowed with the main or most recent physician listed as the contact.

Here is how the student could have written about these three activities in one description:

Dr. Smith, Plastic Surgeon. 1/1/01 - 1/1/02. 300 hrs.
Dr. White, General Surgeon. 1/1/02 - 1/1/03. 100 hrs.
Dr. Jones, Family Medicine. 1/1/03 - 1/1/04. 50 hrs.
These three shadowing experiences gave me more insight into the world of medicine and the daily interactions that physicians have with patients and other health care providers. Seeing how patients were impacted only strengthened my desire to become a physician. (416 characters)

Most Meaningful for the above example:

What made shadowing Dr. Jones so meaningful was the environment and patients. Because of his office location, I was able to see what it was like to care for predominantly lower socioeconomic status patients. I was immensely impacted by how Dr. Jones took his time to get to know his patients, sought to find the best solution or specialty referral that he could at the time for each of them, and worked with them when it came to handling methods of payments for patients with and without insurance. Dr. Jones explained to me that to be a physician you have to desire to serve others through the high points, but especially through the low ones because that is when the patients will need it most. The times I have spent with Dr. Jones have reaffirmed my drive to become a physician and shown me patient care in a whole new light. (829 characters)

I almost always recommend that students stay away from shadowing as a most meaningful experience. Because shadowing is usually a very passive experience, I doubt it is truly meaningful. Don't get me wrong, I remember how exciting it was to shadow—but that is different than meaningful. This student listed one of three shadowing experiences as most meaningful, and you can see that they do a decent job of trying to explain why it was the most meaningful. It would have been even better if they could have told the story of one of the patients that Dr. Jones was able to help. Well-told stories that highlight the impact of an experience will be more meaningful and memorable. On the AMCAS application, you are given 1325 characters for a most meaningful essay, and I recommend you use as many characters as possible for this, as well as all of the other text fields on the application.

Clinical Volunteering

I was able to overcome a cultural and language barrier effectively. It was only a matter of a few days before I felt how many of steps I took forward. My job was to take patients into their rooms, provide them with what they needed, and discharge them by a wheelchair. I learned how to take initiative, to offer help whenever possible, and how much a smile means. I also developed skills to deal with people who have diverse backgrounds, which I enjoyed, and to calm them down when stressed. Initially I was in doubt whether my prosthetic would keep me from pushing wheelchairs for 4 hours. I then discovered that my potential was bigger than this obstacle, and I could perform my job very smoothly. (699 characters)

> *If you're following along, you know this example is filled with the student trying to sell their skills and traits. I don't know who this student is, but I know what they think I want them to be.*

Non-clinical Volunteering

As I struggled to find a single jar of peanut butter that qualified for the food assistance program's strict regulations with "Jerese," a recent Congolese refugee with very limited understanding of English, I got a glimpse of the bravery required to leave home and everything familiar behind. While volunteering with Jerese's family was initially an assignment, our relationship grew into friendship. Whether it was helping find affordable car seats for the kids or cheering for Jerese's husband, "Anjelo," as he scored the winning goal in our local soccer league's championship game, it was rewarding to be able to help the family develop their new life and help them navigate American culture. (695 characters)

> *This example highlights how a story can show compassion, empathy, caring, and much more. The student didn't have to sell any of those things. They didn't go into specific detail about their job duties either. I can see that the student's role was to help integrate an immigrant family, and that's all the reader needs to know.*

Scribe

I scribe patient-provider interactions in the Emergency Room (ER) and facilitate flow and productivity. Each 12-hour shift, I scribe for up to 3 providers prioritizing notes based on urgency and acuity. I developed quick shorthand and learned common medical terminology and diagnoses. Yet each shift is unpredictable with new cases and patients of various backgrounds. For example, in the beginning I trusted every patient only to find out that they were frequent flyers, drug seekers, or inmates wanting food. Each provider has a unique way of interacting with their patients. With constant consults, I observe collaboration between specialties. Understanding the components of a physician note has strengthened my understanding behind patient exams. Despite the long shifts and overload of notes, the problem solving nature and the interactions I see confirms by desire to become a physician. (895 characters *initial draft, over the character count)

> *This is an example of a very generic, job description. The student is describing what a scribe does. Yes, scribes facilitate flow and productivity. They need to develop a shorthand and learn medical terminology. Talking about frequent flyers, drug seekers, and inmates wanting food is negative, which I recommend you avoid. Another very common trend I see in these descriptions is students trying to sell their understanding of medicine or their readiness and skillset necessary to be a medical student or physician—you should avoid this too. This student did this when writing about their understanding of the physical exam.*

Teacher

My lead teacher and I are responsible for 18 seven year olds. I help students navigate through academic, emotional and social challenges. I strive to create a safe environment where kids can establish a routine but also take risks. Using a growth mindset, we emphasize how to think instead of rote memorization of spelling or math facts. I teach a breadth of subjects from math, social studies, literacy. For example, I designed a social studies curriculum around the importance of respecting differences as we explored the social identifiers such as ability, race, gender. On top of managing classroom behavior, we interact with parents on a daily basis or at parent conferences. (680 characters)

> *Hopefully, you've seen the trend already of students writing very generic descriptions. Everything in this description describes what I*

would consider the basic tasks of all teachers. This description gives me no idea of who the student is, which is the goal of the activity section.

Waitress

From high school to present day I have maintained a job as a waitress at Jonny's City Diner. Through this position, I have learned how to engage with, actively listen and effectively communicate with any customer that walks through the doors. This position has taught me how to provide excellent customer service, as well as learn how to capitalize on multitasking, being able to juggle more than one duty at a time. Through this job I have made many relationships through both co-workers and customers and have expanded my connections within my local community. This job has provided me with lifelong memories, skills, relationships and a second family. (655 characters)

You can see this first sentence is wasted characters. The timeline of the position is in the details of the experience and doesn't need to be repeated in the description. Students feel the need to put these details in to lead into the full description, but it is not necessary. This is another example of the student selling communication skills, customer service skills, and other skills the student thinks the Admissions Committee member will be excited to read about. Hopefully, showing you these real examples will give you an idea of how common it is for students to sell themselves. Put yourself in the reviewer's shoes and ask yourself if you would be able to separate applicants when all you have is their "sales pitch."

Sales Clerk

Throughout my high school career and entire college career, I have maintained various jobs while balancing school. One of these jobs was a sales clerk for the Smith's Automotive Group. My job description entailed running a boutique, interacting with customers, providing great customer service, being trusted to handle money and balancing the end of day numbers. All of these roles provided me with a firsthand experience to the business aspect of a large scale company.

Being knowledgeable on the business end of this company encouraged me to pursue a master degree that gave me insight to the business aspects of medicine. (627 characters)

> *This student made it easy to see they were writing about their job description, even specifically using those words in the description. Trying to connect a master's degree to the business aspects of medicine doesn't tell the reader much about why that is important or about the student.*

Scribe

I worked as a medical scribe in a Family Medicine clinic. As a scribe I specialized in medical data entry into the electronic health record system. I improved the medical provider's ability to provide direct patient care. I worked in a fast paced environment and adapted to the needs and methods of various physicians. I became fluent in medical terminology and familiar with the breadth their examination process. I learned that patients cannot always express what is bothering them or answer medical questions and observed how physicians examine patients in a way that makes them cooperative and feel safe. (608 characters)

> *This is another example of a student writing very generic information about being a scribe. The last part of the description is what the student learned. Usually, as soon as I see a statement like "I learned," "I understand," or "This taught me that," I can bet what follows is not important for me to understand the student. What I do know is that students usually write these things to show they think they are ready to be medical students and physicians. A lot of these statements are very generic, such as, "I learned that patients cannot always express what is bothering them or answer medical questions." A statement like this is something that most people know—even those not in or interested in, pursuing medicine.*

Scribe

I was looking for a job that fits my desire of getting more related to medicine. I had the opportunity to work as a medical scribe at a Sports Medicine clinic which I enjoyed. I documented history and symptoms as well as plans of the physician for about 20 patients a day. I have learned how to adapt fast to a new specialty. My continuous questions and research about orthopedics had made me able to follow with the physician as he was diagnosing and treating patients. I also developed more sense of discipline and endurance. For me, being around and with physicians is one of the best ways to get prepared, as a future doctor, with high skills and unique personality. (670 characters)

Here again, you can see the student writing a very generic description about their role as a scribe. The majority of this is to sell the reviewer on the skills they gained.

Here is the same student as above, with another scribe entry:

This was volunteer work that I will cherish forever. I gained this position after proving myself as an exceptional student when I shadowed the physician. My job there was to see patients with the doctor to document their medical history, main complaints and symptoms on eClinicalWorks system. On average, I used to see 7 patients a day. Despite being completely new for me, I succeeded with this job and learned that prosperity comes with making mistakes, asking questions, and being brave enough to face one's fears and obstacles. My success in this experience got me into a new level which is being an employee with ScribeAmerica. (632 characters)

Having multiple entries of the same type of activity is something I wouldn't recommend for most students. Even if you worked at multiple locations or for multiple companies, one scribe activity is usually enough. This student again used the description to talk about the basics of being a scribe and sell their success. One exception to multiple entries for the same type of activity or company would be if you were a scribe (or something else), and then you became a leader for that position. It is very common for students to be promoted from a scribe to the lead scribe. I recommend students put each of these experiences in separate entries, with one as clinical experience and the other as leadership experience.

Most Meaningful for the above example:

"Move, but do not move the way fear makes you move." This was the quote that was echoing in my head when I headed for the first time to the Medical Center to work there as a scribe. I was so afraid of this completely new experience for me. I heard my actual voice saying "go back! Do not do it!" I ignored that voice and forced myself to keep going, refusing to retreat out of fear. I admit that I started as a shy girl trying to survive in this very busy clinic. Gradually, I started to feel, for the first time, a love of medicine, of taking care of patients and listening to their worries. This true love grew to a deep passion which exposed my inner strength. I did not hold back any effort that would help the clinic. Specifically, I focused on being on time, performing my work quickly and effectively, dealing with patients very professionally and interacting kindly with my colleagues. The biggest challenge for me was that I was the youngest there. I had to prove myself and exceed their expectations. I learned from every experience every day. Many residents rotating there were amazed by my work! I was very proud when my supervising doctor told me "you started as a shy girl, and now you are very strong and confident." (1253 characters)

This student is very focused on the sales pitch, which is why I wanted to include this example. After discussing this with the student, they could really see the impact of focusing more on the story. Do you think that being "focused on being on time, performing my work quickly and effectively, dealing with patients very professionally and interacting kindly with my colleagues" is something that will set you apart? Don't be like most students and think the traits you are trying to sell are unique to you.

Research Assistant

As a high school volunteer in Dr. Pearse's lab, I collected data for an ongoing experiment that continued for another two years, during which I came in on my breaks from college to finish the data collection. Based on this performance, in 2016 I received an NIH grant to continue my work in the lab while participating in their Neurotrauma Summer Research Internship Program. Of hundreds of applicants, eleven students were given the opportunity to learn from lectures and journal clubs as well as to conduct their own study. My final poster was titled "Examining the Tolerability of Cell Transplant Doses in an Experimental Rodent Model of Chronic Spinal Cord Injury". (665 characters)

Can you tell me the goal of this activity description? The activity is for a research assistant, but the description is mostly around winning an award. Remember that you don't need to "sell" how awesome you are. For the AACOMAS and TMDSAS applications, you have space to include the award separately. For AMCAS, you should focus more on yourself and your impact on the research through a story, and just very briefly mention the award. The poster title for AMCAS would take up too much space and doesn't matter here. I would mention the award and poster briefly to keep room for more of the story.

Executive Board, Event Coordinator

Initially drawn to this organization because of my passion for aiding underserved immigrant populations and tutoring children, my high-level involvement in just a few months lead to my election to the executive board. This position allowed me to help provide opportunities in education and empowerment for children affected by social injustice in Latin America as well as similar opportunities for immigrant children in Gainesville. Specifically, I was tasked with organizing all philanthropic and social events, recruiting new members, and raising awareness on campus. The largest event I organized was a "Zumbathon," in which we danced for three hours to raised money for the cause. (684 characters)

As the reviewer starts to read this example, they are immediately hit with the sales pitch of being passionate about aiding the underserved immigrant population and tutoring children. Let the activity do the selling for you. Let the story show your passion without needing to say it. The last sentence could have been turned into the story of organizing this event and the impact it had. How much money was raised? How many people danced? How many lives will be positively affected by the money raised?

Club Membership

As a Hispanic woman, being a part of the Latino Student Association at my university helped me grow closer and better understand my Mexican culture as well as the culture of many other students with family from many Latin American countries. In meetings, we not only learned about all the different countries and cultures, but we also planned fundraiser and service events to spread those cultures throughout the campus. Some events would be Taco Tuesday fundraisers or Getting to Know Hispanics Q&A. (500 characters)

I wanted to include this example because many of you are members of clubs—not on an executive committee or some sort of leadership committee, but just a member. When you are "just" a member of a club, similar to shadowing, there usually isn't anything impactful that you will extract from that activity to discuss in your application. Depending on their level of involvement, this student could have talked about how they impacted the fundraiser events.

Resident Assistant/Community Advisor

A Community Advisor (CA) is an individual that is part of the Department of Residence at State University. As a CA, I worked in the apartment community with around one hundred and fifteen students per semester. I provided resources and events for students to deal with a wide variety of problems, including issues adapting to life in our state or the United States or issues with academics. I had the pleasure of watching friendships form at community events I planned and watching students' grades increase from resources I suggested, but I believe my most impactful interactions centered around my resident's mental health and helping them access the resources they needed. (675 characters)

> *Many students are RAs or CAs. It's a great opportunity to show leadership, communication skills, and more. Remember that the goal of these descriptions is not to sell yourself or write a basic job description but instead, tell a story. This description is generic and could be copied and pasted into another student's application. Reading a story of the student interacting with some of the residents and handling a difficult situation would show everything that is needed.*

Resident Assistant/Community Advisor

During the demanding year of being an RA of 55 residents, I was faced with many challenges that blurred the lines between a friend and an RA. I had always gotten along with my suitemates and often got food together; however, one night walking by their room I saw a suitcase full of beer. This became a challenge for me knowing that writing them up was going to infringe on our relationship, yet it was policy and less drastic than a police ticket for underage drinking. I wrote them up and explained why I had to do that. They weren't happy about it but understood why. Eventually, I became more comfortable with the role and its strain as I got better at walking that line with all of my residents. (699 characters)

> *You can see the difference between this description and the previous one. The former was a basic description of every RA's role. This description goes into a story of a dilemma this student faced and the thought process behind the resolution. This shows me who the student is, while the previous one does not.*

Fitness Instructor

As a group fitness instructor, I was tasked with the responsibility of designing and executing weekly fitness classes for patrons of all physical and health conditions. Depending on the patron and any limitations they may have had, I provided modifications for all exercises. I also attended teamwork development meetings with coworkers to better improve our own classes as well as provide constructive feedback for each other. Being a lead trainer, I was given the opportunity to train new instructors and further develop my leadership skills. (544 characters)

I included this activity because of what the student wrote about and how they classified this experience—Paid Employment - Not Medical/ Clinical. At its core, it is a basic job description. The student wrote about being the lead trainer, though. I would have thought about adding this under the heading of Leadership. There isn't anything magical about having paid employment on an application, and if this was listed under Leadership, it would have been easy to see it was a paid job. For the description, if listed under Leadership, the student could have included a story of helping a new instructor who was struggling. This would have shown the leadership, compassion, teamwork, and communication skills—all from one story.

Volunteer Medical Assistant

As a clinical volunteer, I greeted and prepared patients to be seen by physicians, as well as assisted nurses with recording weight, vital signs and medical history. This experience taught me about care of underserved and geriatric patients and allowed me to practice this care in Spanish and English. Even more valuable were my interactions with French speaking patients who had immigrated to Miami because of the 2010 earthquake in Haiti. As I do not speak French, this experience challenged me to communicate with the few words I do know and a little help from Google Translate until an interpreter was available. Most importantly, I learned the value nonverbal communication with patients. (691 characters)

I would be interested to see how this activity was classified. I'm assuming it was classified as a clinical/medical experience even though the student does a good job of telling us at the beginning that it likely wasn't clinical experience and was probably more clerical or administrative. I read the part about assisting the nurses with recording details as data entry and not actually weighing the patient and taking the vital signs. Be careful not to throw yourself under the bus by taking what may be a perfectly good clinical experience and making it sound like it's not. Most people know what a medical assistant does, so writing about the job description isn't necessary. Save those characters for telling the story of an interaction with your most memorable patient. This is another example of the student writing a lot about a learning experience, which doesn't tell the reader anything about the student.

Circuit Court Judge Campaign Volunteer

As an intern on this campaign I was primarily tasked with promoting the candidate in Spanish-speaking senior centers throughout the country. In addition, my team and were assigned small businesses, festivals, and other special events. This experience allowed me to explore unique cultural neighborhoods in my own home city and interact with immigrants from complex and rich cultural backgrounds, who were always eager to share their stories. Although this experience is very different from the career I decided to pursue, I appreciate that it allowed me to communicate with a diverse range of communities. (605 characters)

The student could have shared a great story interacting with people at the senior centers, showing their ability to communicate without selling the reader on how the activity allowed them to communicate. A good story will always be stronger than the sales pitch. I can tell that the point of this description is to show the student has the ability to interact with a diverse set of people, hoping the reader can see they will be good at interacting with patients who come from diverse backgrounds. Can you see that too?

Hobby/Rock Climbing

As someone who requires a physical outlet to destress, climbing has become a huge part of my life outside of work. I specifically enjoy approaching a problem or route that requires me to think critically about how to approach the wall. I enjoy evaluating where to place my hands and feet while also being conscious of what I am physically capable of. It is also important to calculate the risk of each move and the possible outcome of falling. After I plan the route I enjoy focusing on executing the necessary moves. It is a great way for me to clear my head and allow me to continue to set and accomplish goals outside of my pursuit of medicine. (647 characters)

I love putting hobbies in the activity section. Usually, students only have space for one or two entries to talk about hobbies. The goal of putting in your most significant hobby is to show who you are as a person outside of all of the premed craziness. Unfortunately, what this student did was take their hobby and use it as a sales pitch for what they think is important to being a physician—the ability to think critically. This defeats the purpose of showing the reviewer who they are; all the student is doing is showing the reviewer what the student thinks the med schools want to read about.

EMT

As an EMT Basic, I worked for a 911 transport service. I responded to emergency calls and provided immediate care under the supervision of a paramedic. At times I also completed transfers between facilities. I was responsible for maintaining supplies and tools on the ambulance. Prior to being an EMT Basic I did not have any patient care experience. I developed assessment skills, patient interaction skills, and advanced life support assistance skills. In addition to developing clinical skills I also gained perspective on how the healthcare setting operates in general. (573 characters)

If you don't know what an EMT is or what they do, raise your hand. Out of 1,000 reviewers, my guess is that no one would raise their hand. The majority of this description talks about what an EMT does. The student would have done a much more effective job by telling an impactful story of treating a patient as an EMT. You can see from the last sentence that the student is trying to show they understand healthcare from this experience. Many students think the goal of the application is to prove you understand what you are getting yourself into. I would argue that this is exactly what the application is for, but instead of telling the reader you understand healthcare, you need to show it through the stories of your experiences.

EMT

The car was upside-down in the ditch as we arrived on the scene. I helped my paramedic carry supplies to the patient, stabilize his head, and attach the backboard. I assisted as we re-assessed the patient in the ambulance and drove quickly to the nearest hospital so he could be flown by helicopter to a bigger hospital. Experiences like these taught me a lot about medicine as an emergency medical technician. I also received my first exposure to patient care and emergency medicine within a rural community, where I learned of the unique issues that rural communities face compared to urban areas, such as lower access to physicians and the higher incidence of disease that can follow. (687 characters)

In this EMT example, the student started off really well—they were telling a story. They should have finished the story instead of switching to their exposure to rural medicine and what they learned. Think about it this way: Will an Admissions Committee member say, "Hey—we finally found someone who knows the unique issues that rural communities face because they said it right here in their application!!!" No, they won't. With one tweak of a sentence—adding a bit about being in a rural setting as they arrived on the scene, the reader could extrapolate that the student has exposure to rural communities.

Conference Attendance

While attending the patient congress I met "Ann," an incredible woman battling multiple sclerosis. She traveled to D.C. to share the challenges she endured with the foundation members, so she could raise awareness of palliative care in the management of chronic illnesses. She sat next to me, hands shaking as she told the story of her diagnosis and loss of her job. She choked up as she spoke of raising her daughter while managing appointments with multiple specialists. As her disease progressed, she battled to maintain control of her body and life. Her passion inspired me to share my own story with my representatives to advocate for the Palliative Care and Hospice Education and Training Act. (699 characters)

> *A lot of students attend conferences and usually write very simple things like interacting and networking with physicians or going to sessions and poster presentations and learning. Instead, this student did a great job of telling the story of an interaction with a patient. This example helps the reader see the student interacting with the patient and displaying compassion—something the student did not have to sell to get across.*

Child Life

One Saturday I was sent to the room of a 3-month-old surgical patient. I sat holding the tiny baby closely watching the monitor for any signs of distress. A technician came to perform an EKG while I held the baby's fragile sleeping body. I gently unfolded the swaddle exposing the babies arms and chest so the technician could attach the leads. He squirmed slightly, but with some quit hushes he settled and allowed the tech to complete the test. Then two doctors came in to conduct an exam. They pushed on his abdomen and listened to his heart and lungs. As I sat holding the baby I couldn't help but wonder how challenging such exams must be without a volunteer or family member in the room. (693 characters)

Child Life is a very popular activity for premed students. Many students try to focus on the skills and traits they have to be successful as a Child Life volunteer and how that carries over to being a physician. In truth, you should avoid any and all comparisons to medicine and being a physician in your descriptions. Here, instead, this student does a great job of telling a story. The one change I would make to this would be to give the baby a name. Names are more memorable than "the baby." You might read this and think it doesn't do a good job of explaining what the student learned, or what skills they have that are going to make a great physician—that is exactly why I think it's a great activity description. It only needs to tell a story of who you are, not how great you think you are.

Orientation Leader

Following one of the multiple orientation events on college parties, I sat with my group to discuss the presentation. The students sat quietly looking at the ground unwilling to talk. I looked at my co-orientation leader and we both immediately knew we had to do something to change the mood. To break the ice, I started telling a story of how I had protected a friend in a dangerous situation at a recent party. As I opened up, so did the students in my group. One by one they began sharing stories of different situations they had been in where they or someone they knew had been in a challenging situation. We worked as a group to come up with useful strategies for de-escalation. (683 characters)

Being an orientation leader is another common activity for students. A bad example would include a sales pitch about leadership skills, communication skills, or organizational skills. Here, this student did a great job of avoiding the sales pitch and instead focused on the story.

Fundraising

Over the course of 4 years, I helped my school raise over $160,000 for the American Cancer Society through Relay for Life events. The teams I captained raised just under $5,000, and I personally raised $1,790 over 4 years. I joined the Relay planning committee during my sophomore year as the entertainment chair. During my sophomore and junior years, I organized entertainment for 7 different fundraising events. My senior year I acted as the senior advisor to the planning committee and helped organize my last Relay. Some of my favorite memories from my undergrad were made participating in Relay for Life. (609 characters)

> *Fundraising is a very common activity for students, whether through organizations such as Relay for Life, Dance Marathon, or even fraternities and sororities. I like to have the student focus on impact. The impact of these types of activities can be shown through numbers. You can see in this example the student did a great job showing how much money was raised both individually and as a group. This shows great leadership and impact, which gives the Admissions Committees insight into the student.*

Music

As a French horn player for University Symphony Orchestra, I perform with the orchestra several times each semester. Before rehearsals, I am expected to research and practice pieces of music so I can play my part accurately the first time we rehearse as a group. During rehearsals, I listen carefully to the other French horn players so we can match pitches, styles, and articulations. Daily practice and strict regimens are required to maintain the level of performance needed to work with the orchestra. I was recently named a finalist in the Concerto Competition where musicians compete for four spots to perform as soloists with the University Orchestra and plan to compete again next year. (696 characters)

> *Music is a great extracurricular, and depending on what you did, it could be a hobby, volunteering, leadership, or something else. You can see from this example that the student took a very light activity and tried to sell it very hard. Using a story, I would have suggested the student write about a time they played in a concert—what did*

they feel as they stared out into the crowd? Instead, the student tried to sell working hard and dedication. Anyone will know that if you're playing at the university orchestra level and you were named a finalist in a competition, you have to have a certain level of dedication—you don't have to sell this.

PERSONAL STATEMENT

The personal statement is one of the first things that students face off with during the medical school application cycle. Sitting in front of a blank screen for hours on end is a scary, and oftentimes, anxiety-provoking exercise. I've talked to many students who delay applying to medical school only because they didn't want to write their personal statement.

I wrote a whole book about the personal statement—I highly recommend you check out *The Premed Playbook: Guide to the Medical School Personal Statement*. It has helped thousands of premeds (and other pre-health students) figure out how to start planning for their personal statement, figure out what to write about, learn how to write it, and most importantly, learn what mistakes to avoid.

In this book, I'll cover some very important pieces of the personal statement that you need to be aware of to make sure you don't make the most common mistakes that could put your application in the trash can.

What is the Goal of the Personal Statement?

When I'm working with students who are struggling with the personal statement, one of the first questions I ask them is, "What do you think is the goal of the personal statement?" More often than not, they get this question wrong.

The goal of the personal statement is to show the Admissions Committee why you want to be a physician. I repeat this statement over and over and over again in our Facebook Hangout group (premedhangout.com), during my Facebook Live videos, on Instagram, and in my podcast episodes, yet time and time again, I get questions from students asking me if they should write about a certain situation. I follow up their question with another question: "How does this situation, this experience, make you want to be a physician?"

An experience may be very impactful in your life, but if it is not guiding you toward being a physician, then you probably shouldn't write about it. If an experience is showing the reader that you are great with people, then you are not writing a personal statement—you are writing an argumentative paper about why you think you are going to be a great physician because of your "people skills." A lot of students make the mistake of trying to show the reader why they're going to be a good physician or why they think they understand what being in medicine is like, and therefore, why they are *ready* to enter medicine. Students even talk about what they view as the negative aspects of medicine and how, in spite of those things, they still want to be a physician.

These are not things you need to write about in your personal statement. Your personal statement should focus on your initial experiences around when you decided and started exploring the idea of healthcare. This is what I call your "seed." Your seed doesn't have to point to being a physician. If you started out wanting to be a nurse, physical therapist, veterinarian, or something else related to healthcare, that is still your seed. If you did go down one of those paths, you'll need to switch gears at some point to explain why you want to be a physician now.

Your personal statement should discuss the experiences you've had that have reaffirmed why you want to be a physician. I call these experiences your "watering of the seed" moments. You have your seed, and then you have what watered your seed. That is what the bulk of your personal statement should be about.

If an Admissions Committee member is reading a personal statement and can see the student doesn't truly understand what they are getting into, or they are potentially chasing after this dream for the wrong reasons and will not be happy being a physician, it is likely the medical school will not want to take a chance on that student—even with great stats.

I spoke to a student recently who had a 3.9 GPA and a 519 MCAT score. They didn't get in anywhere. They didn't even get a single interview. Why? Because they completely lacked any real exposure to medicine. The student had zero clinical experience and zero shadowing. If you don't know what you are getting yourself into, medical schools don't want to risk it. As soon as you realize that medical school and being a physician is not what you thought it was going to be like, you are likely going to bail, at best; at worst, you will continue on the path and become a toxic classmate and a toxic resident.

There is a glorification of physicians in the media, especially in TV shows. It seems like every year, there is at least one new medical drama. Admissions Committees want to make sure you want to be a physician for the *right* reasons and not just because you grew up watching "Scrubs" and "Grey's Anatomy."

Being Cliché?

All of us, at some point in our life, have had some exposure to medicine. The most common exposure that we have is either through an ill or injured family member or being ill or injured ourselves. This is oftentimes the first exposure to healthcare and the experience that piqued your interest to want to further explore medicine—your "seed."

Having that story is not cliché. It is *your story*. It would be cliché to say you want to be a doctor because you want to help people. There is no story there. This is not your path—those are just empty words. I was at a meetup recently, and a student asked a question about how common it is to talk about illness. They asked, "Aren't medical schools desensitized to the story of your grandmother getting sick or your dad getting injured?" It was easy for me to respond with, "Absolutely not!"

What medical schools are desensitized to is students writing personal statements about how they are motivated, dedicated, hardworking, empathetic, and compassionate. They are tired of students trying to sell them on their great communication skills, as if those alone will make them become amazing physicians.

What medical schools, and humans, will never be desensitized to are stories they can connect with. Schools can never become desensitized to the story of how you were affected by your dad getting injured or your grandmother becoming ill. We're wired to be attracted to and connect with those stories, assuming you write them well.

So, as you are thinking about what to write about, don't think about it from the standpoint of, "How do I prove that I'm going to be a great physician?" Think about it from another point of view: "How do I tell my story of how I got to this point?" Highlight diverse experiences that have exposed you to medicine, patients, and physicians—experiences that have encouraged you, motivated you, and reassured you that this is the right path for you. That is what you need to write about in your personal statement.

Any reader should be able to finish your personal statement and say, "Okay, I understand why Sally wants to be a doctor. I understand when they were first exposed to medicine. I understand what they've been doing since to continue, to confirm in their mind, and to reassure us as an admissions committee that they want to be a physician."

Again, don't worry about whether your experiences are common. Don't avoid telling your story in an attempt to be different.

How Important is the Personal Statement?

Like most aspects of the medical school application, it depends. How each med school uses the personal statement can vary widely. How one school uses it in their admissions process will look completely different than another. Some schools will place a lot of weight on a personal statement to determine if a student will get an interview—other schools may use the student's secondary essay answers more heavily.

The most important thing to remember with the personal statement, and any other part of the admissions process, is that you cannot control how the Admissions Committee is going to view your personal statement, activities list, secondaries, etc. All you can do is put your best foot forward and hope they like it and think you're a good fit.

When Should I Start the Personal Statement?

If there is one thing I know for sure, it is that the personal statement takes much more time to write than most students think. For that reason, I recommend starting your drafting process in January of the year you are going to apply to medical school (the year before you're planning on starting medical school).

That will give you enough time to brainstorm ideas about your personal statement, to think about everything you have experienced on your journey, and to decide what you want to write about. Then you'll have to actually write the essay, get feedback, take time away to get fresh eyes, and hopefully finish it with time to spare.

Most premed students seem to be type-A students and think they are going to sit down in one session and come out with a polished, perfectly edited personal statement that they can copy and paste right into the application. Do not make this your goal. Your goal is to write a terrible first draft. Then write a slightly less terrible second draft. Continue this process over and over again, and you'll get to where you need to be.

The actual preparation for the personal statement can, and should, start much sooner. Hopefully, you're journaling your thoughts and emotions after each of your experiences. These journal entries will come in very handy when you start writing your first draft of your personal statement. I've talked to too many students who have forgotten what they did just a few years ago. Don't let this be you.

How Long Can the Personal Statement Be?

The personal statement can only be 5,300 characters (including spaces) for AMCAS and AACOMAS. For TMDSAS, the essay length is only 5,000 characters. I recommend trying to be at or above 5,000 characters for AMCAS and AACOMAS. Anything shorter, and it looks a little awkward.

Do I Need to Write Separate Personal Statements for Each Application Service?

Other than TMDSAS being 300 characters shorter than AMCAS and AACOMAS, there aren't any major differences in what you should be writing about in your personal statement, so you don't need different ones if you are applying to multiple application services.

Remember, the personal statement is sent to every school that you designate in your application. If you have 15 schools designated, all 15 schools are going to get the exact same essay. You cannot personalize the personal statement to each school.

If you're applying to an Early Decision program school, you should still write a general personal statement in case you don't get accepted and need to add other schools later.

If you have specific reasons to only be applying to one school (not just Early Decision), you can personalize it in that case.

What Makes a Great Personal Statement?

When I'm a few sentences into a personal statement, I usually know whether or not it is going to be great, okay, or terrible. Any personal statement that starts with "I knew from a young age that I wanted to be a doctor" is a recipe for disaster.

When I talk about how you need to write your story, I really mean that it should be a story. It should take the reader on your journey. They should be able to see what you saw—feel what you felt. You do this by using a very common writing technique called *showing* instead of *telling*. If you do a quick Google search of "show vs. tell," you'll see a ton of great examples to help guide you to better writing. The more you can engage the senses of the reader, the better your storytelling and your personal statement will be.

The opening should involve some of the most engaging parts of your personal statement to *hook* the reader and make them want to keep reading. Think of every sentence and every paragraph having a job—to get the reader to keep reading. The personal statement does not have to be in chronological order—it does not need to go from seed to watering. If you have an experience later on in your journey that you think would make for an interesting opening, try that. Remember, you'll be going through a lot of drafts, so try something and see how it works. If you don't like it, you'll just need to write another draft.

Be careful, though. *Showing* can oftentimes go too far into the creative writing space. The personal statement is not a creative writing piece.

Check out this example of showing vs. telling from a student's personal statement:

Telling: I woke up one morning to my mother crying as she frantically told me that my grandmother was being rushed into the ER.
Showing: Frantic crying and screaming was my alarm clock the morning I found out my grandmother was being rushed to the ER.

Great personal statements *show* the reader your journey. By the end, they can *feel* why you want to be a doctor. They were there with you when you were at the hospital seeing your father die. They were there with you when you volunteered at the hospital for the first time and interacted with your first patient. They can see why this is what you want to do.

Reflection—a.k.a. The Takeaway

I could have added this to the previous point of what makes a personal statement great, but I felt like it needed its own section.

One of the biggest mistakes students make when writing the personal statement is focusing too much on the *what* and not enough on the *why*. You can do everything right—paint a picture of your seed and the experiences that have strengthened your desire to be a physician—but if you fail to connect those experiences with *why* they made you want to explore healthcare or confirmed that being a physician was right for you, then you're missing the point of the personal statement.

Reflecting on each experience is key to telling the reader *why* that experience you just showed them was important.

Each takeaway should ideally be focused on why it strengthened your desire to be a doctor—not that it taught you something about being a physician or some other generic takeaway.

Check out these two examples that talk more about the *what* instead of the *why* despite experiences that should have led to why the experience strengthened their desire to be a physician:

"I was reminded that as a physician, I wish to approach the patient and the varying facets of medicine from a place of holism."

> *Writing about how you want to treat patients doesn't tell the reader why you want to be a physician.*

"I know and desire to work as a physician in underserved communities."

> *Writing about the types of patients you want to treat doesn't help the reader understand why you want to be a physician.*

"At this moment, I realized human health and illness seemed to draw my attention."

> *Being nonspecific about what it is you want can lead the reader to see you in many different positions. Having your attention drawn to human health and illness doesn't mean you need to be a physician.*

"I knew at that moment I wanted to do more for that patient than just hand over a defibrillator and watch from the outside."

> *This takeaway came after a good experience showing the student interacting with a patient and other members of the healthcare team. The takeaway is focusing on wanting to do more. It's a good takeaway. This is a very common takeaway, especially for those who are coming from being in healthcare already. Since writing my personal statement book, I've definitely seen more of this type of takeaway. Be careful with it, and don't just generically say that you want to do more—try to focus on why you want to do more.*

How to Conclude Your Personal Statement

Wrapping up your personal statement is just as important as hooking the reader at the beginning. A very common conclusion—one I think you should avoid—is the "summary" type of conclusion. Students will show the reader a couple of great experiences and then summarize those experiences in the conclusion. Doing this is just repeating what you've already talked about. It's a waste of the limited characters that you are given in your personal statement.

It's a very common "English 101" type format, as well as a presentation format:

Intro: Tell them what you are going to tell them

Body: Tell them

Conclusion: Tell them what you told them

This is *not* how to write your personal statement.

I think one of the main goals of your conclusion is to try to highlight what you hope to accomplish as a physician. After you have shown the reader why you want to be a doctor, you can conclude with what you are going to do with the diploma that the school is going to give you. How are you going to make them proud?

Here's an example of a summary conclusion:

"Amid the chaos of the country club, a seemingly offbeat incident paved a pathway to medicine. The strain my father and uncle experienced from the lack of awareness about healthcare confirmed my decision to give back to the underserved community. As I step out of the clinic every week, a new patient's story becomes part of my own and inspires me to work clinically for the medically disadvantaged. Each experience has developed a passion in me to not only grasp the knowledge required to clinically diagnose an individual but also commit to the greater purpose of giving back to one's community."

In contrast, here's an example of a student talking about what they hope to accomplish:

"As a physician, I want to be both a source of knowledge but also a source of relief to my future patients. I hope to look back on my career knowing that I went above and beyond for each patient in an effort to provide them the best standard of care possible. The patients I have connected with thus far have each reminded me of the feeling of hope and lightness I felt leaving that doctor's office when I was 7. They inspire me to pay it forward by becoming a doctor to help future patients as the previous ones have helped me. It is both the fond memories of old patients and the vibrant visions of future patients that make it impossible for me to be anything but a physician."

Who Should Edit my Personal Statement?

Your personal statement, ideally, should be edited by someone with knowledge of what the personal statement is, and its purpose. If you have access to a premed advisor on your campus, you should start there. Hopefully, they have enough experience to give you some great feedback.

Many students turn to physician mentors, current medical students, and other premeds for advice. You can use these people to give you feedback but remember that just because a physician or medical student got into medical school, doesn't mean they necessarily know what makes a good personal statement and how to give great feedback.

I created a review sheet that you can give to editors to make sure they understand the type of feedback they should be giving you. I included it in my personal statement book, and you can have it, too. Go to personalstatementbook. com/reviewsheet to download our "Guide to Reviewing Personal Statements."

Additionally, you can use the Premed Hangout Facebook group (premed-hangout.com) and ask other students there if they will look at your personal statement.

You can also use paid services, if that is something you want to do, as well. I wrote *The Premed Playbook: Guide to the Medical School Personal Statement* so no one needs to use a service to get feedback on their personal statement, but some students still want a little bit of extra help, and that's why we offer those services as well. You can find out how to work with our Mappd team at editmyps.com.

Grammar

I highly encourage you to use the service Grammarly as you are writing your personal statement. I'm using it right now for one last pass on this book. It not only helps with typos, but it also helps with sentence structure and much more.

You can use this for your personal statement, but it will also help with anything you are writing, including emails to professors for letters of recommendation, your activity descriptions, and much more. It is a free service, but I recommend the premium version, at least until you finish your secondary essays.

Check out Grammarly for free to start at https://medicalschoolhq.net/grammarly. (Using that link will give me a small affiliate commission if you decide to sign up.)

Grammarly plugs directly into your browser, Microsoft Word, and to Google Docs, so it is there to help you wherever you are writing.

What Should I Avoid in my Personal Statement?

You may think that my "seed and watering of the seed" framework makes for generic personal statements, but it doesn't. It gives you the flexibility to write about your experiences and tell your story. I want to make sure you are focusing on the right parts of your story.

While you are concentrating on your story, there are many things you should try to avoid in your personal statement. I have a lot more of these, and I dig into them a lot more in-depth in my personal statement book, *The Premed Playbook: Guide to the Medical School Personal Statement*, but here are some key things to avoid.

Negativity

No one likes a negative person. They just aren't very fun to be around. The Admissions Committee is trying to put together a community of students who will be working very closely together for the next four years. They will likely stay away from a student who comes across as negative in a personal statement.

You may not be aware of a negative comment, but they happen a lot. Talking about your doctor or your family member's doctor, and how they missed a diagnosis or didn't treat you well is not something that you should write about.

You may be a minority who is underrepresented in medicine and have an experience highlighting how that underrepresentation affected a patient, and you want to talk about that experience because you can then show that you want to fix that problem. Don't do this. All you are doing in this situation is being negative towards the current reality of the situation. There are ways to focus on the positive and what you hope to accomplish without bringing up the negative.

Instead of talking about how your mom was misdiagnosed and suffered because of what you perceived to be an uncaring doctor, focus on your mom's diagnosis and how you want to be there for patients like her in the future. This allows you to show you are focused on caring for patients without bringing up negativity.

Résumé

Your personal statement should not be an essay form of your résumé. It is not the place to focus on *everything* you've done. Your activities list, which is part of your application, is the place to list your experiences. The specific and most meaningful experiences that have led you to want to be a physician, your *seed* and *watering of the seed experiences* are what you want to focus on in your personal statement.

The best way to prepare for your applications is to journal your experiences. Every time you shadow, have clinical experience, or any other experiences, whether it is paid or not, you should be journaling. Don't just write about what you did, but what you experienced and how it made you feel. For experiences with patients, ask yourself the question: "Why did this further strengthen my desire to be a physician?"

The platform that I co-founded, Mappd, allows you to track everything you do and journal about it as well. Sign up for a free two-week trial at Mappd.com.

Here is an example of a résumé type experience:

"After a year at the nursing facility, I found a job at the hospital. While I was sad to leave my patients at the nursing facility, I was ready to work in a more acute environment. I started as a medical assistant on the cardiology floor, and after a year of working there, my role is now a Cardiac Cath Technician in the Cath Lab."

This example is just giving the reader a timeline of the student's path without giving the reader any information about why the experiences were important to the student or why they motivated them to continue down this path.

Research

This is probably the most controversial of all. I tell students to avoid writing about research in the personal statement. You may love research and have a lot of experience in it, and you may want to continue doing research as part of your career; if this is the case, then focus on this as part of *what* you want to do as a physician, rather than *why* you want to be a physician.

When I see a student focusing on research in a personal statement, I wonder if they have enough clinical experience to highlight why they want to be a doctor or if they are more interested in research than patient care.

Your research will get enough exposure in the activities list—I believe it should stay out of your personal statement.

Even if you are applying to MD/PhD programs through AMCAS, you should avoid writing about your prior research in your personal statement. You'll have two additional essays in your application to write about your research. Your personal statement should still stay focused on your seed and watering of the seed experiences.

Emotional Topics

Remember that anything in your application is fair game for your interviews. If you think you'll be safe writing about a topic that would normally bring you to tears, you need to make sure you're going to be comfortable talking about it during an interview as well. A few tears during an interview are not the worst thing that can happen, but if you get too emotional, it may hurt your chances of getting an acceptance.

Disabilities and Mental Health

This is a complicated topic. You would think that medical schools would be welcoming to students who have had their own health struggles, both physical and mental, because it would help them understand their future patients.

Unfortunately, Admissions Committees have to weigh everything against whether or not you are going to be able to complete medical school in four years. In the back of their minds, they may also be thinking about the accommodations they will have to provide not only during the preclinical years in the classroom and for tests, but also for your clinical years in the hospital and clinics. Unfortunately, some Admissions Committee members may have some implicit or explicit bias towards those with mental health histories or disabilities.

If your own health journey isn't a significant part of why you want to be a physician, then it doesn't need to be part of your personal statement. Remember, the personal statement is all about why you want to be a physician.

At the end of the day, I need you to be you and tell your story—especially if that past health history is a significant reason for why you want to be a physician. You have to be true to who you are. Just understand there are some who will read your personal statement and pass on offering you an interview because of it.

Trust and Thanks

When I'm reading a personal statement, and I see comments about trust and thanks, I get concerned. I start to think that the student wants to be a doctor to be trusted or to be thanked by their patients. Medicine is so much more than the relationships and trust you earn as a physician. Yes, you need the patient's trust to provide the best care, but that shouldn't be your driving force.

Here are some examples:

"…cannot think of anything more rewarding than having patients place their trust in you during their most vulnerable times."

"She took my hands and continuously thanked me. While I didn't feel as if I had done much, her gratitude washed over me."

"I knew that I wanted to become a physician to accomplish a level of trust."

Students love to write about patients thanking them or the physicians they are shadowing. What happens when you are working as a physician, and the majority of patients you see do not thank you? What will happen then? If that is a big factor in your decision to be a physician (or at least big enough to be included in your personal statement), then I'm going to worry that you are going to be unhappy with your career because you're not receiving the gratitude you expected when you started out on this journey.

Liking Science and Wanting to Help People

We talked a little bit earlier about how most students are on this path because of similar experiences. That's not cliché—that is just common.

That said, writing about liking science or wanting to help people are the two most cliché reasons you can write about in your personal statement.

Helping people can be achieved in any career field. A sanitation worker helps people by taking their trash and recycling. A taxi driver helps people by taking them where they need to go. A financial advisor helps people by getting their retirement savings set up to enjoy their post-work life. You don't need to be a physician to help people.

The same goes for liking science. Just because you like science doesn't mean you should be a physician. You can be a high school science teacher or get your PhD in your preferred scientific field and teach at a medical school. We all have to like science "enough" to get through to be a successful premed and medical student. You definitely do not have to *love* science to be a great physician.

I have seen 1,001 different variations, some very creative, of students trying to show that they like science. I've also seen many variations of students showing that they want to help people. And when you combine liking science and wanting to help people, for some reason, students think that's the magical equation for wanting to be a physician. Believe me—it is not. Avoid it.

Dialog

Maybe it's because I never read a lot growing up, but dialog in a personal statement seems out of place and too hard to follow. Admissions Committee members are reading a lot of essays, and anything that slows them down or confuses them may cause them to lose interest and move on.

Dialog adds confusion. Who's talking? Who are they talking to? Why am I reading this?

It's usually very easy to keep the same meaning and message by changing dialog into non-dialog writing.

Transferring to the Application

You will likely hear from advisors and other students that you shouldn't copy directly from Word or Google Docs and paste directly into the application. I recommend that as well. Oftentimes, hidden characters can throw off formatting that you can't see. The application services could likely fix this on their end, but to be safe, use an online "plain text" editor. A quick Google search led me to editpad.org, which worked perfectly. Mac and Windows operating systems have built-in text editors if you want to use those as well.

Personal Statement Examples

Students supplied the following personal statements that I included in this book. Personal details were changed as much as possible to keep them anonymous. These were not picked to show perfect examples of personal statements—they are good examples of common essays that students turn in for my feedback, which is provided between each paragraph.

Personal Statement 1

Trekking through the gravel on a burning day in Madurai, my fellow students and I reached a colony in the rural outskirts of India. The colony was littered with yellow huts smaller than my freshman dorm room. From a distance, I saw men in white tunics and women in cotton saris going about their day wringing out washed clothes or sweeping up debris outside their home entrances. Spotting us, they instinctively dropped everything and rushed toward us. I could see what leprosy had done to them physically, but where were their spouses? Children? Grandchildren? What immediately struck me was that each person approached us in isolation, without a sign of family ties or kinship. I spotted an elderly lady in a lovely lavender sari leaning on a bamboo stick in a corner, alone. With the attending physician's permission, I walked up to her and greeted her, "Namaste!" She grinned and shook her head bashfully.

This opening has a lot of great showing details but ultimately doesn't seem to lead anywhere. It's over 900 characters of setup. I've seen the best essays use each paragraph to show each part of the story with the reflection at the end of the paragraph, so each paragraph is a self-contained part of the student's journey. With this opening, the reader has to keep reading to figure out what is going on, but at this point, you may lose their interest. We also don't see any hints of medicine other than that these people had leprosy.

I tried to speak the few Tamil words I learned on the trip. She responded in Hindi, "I don't speak Tamil. Can you understand?" Luckily enough, I did. I had been learning Hindi for the past two years to expand my knowledge on South Asian linguistics, beyond the Bangla I grew up learning. I had only dreamed of speaking it abroad. Our conversation flowed in her native tongue. I asked what life was like in the colony. She told me heart-rending tales of how inhabitants of that community had ended up there, when their families abandoned them to save their "reputations". These people had nowhere to turn because they were now "untouchables". I was shattered. Growing up as a South Asian, I was always taught that dignity is defined by humility and looking beyond oneself to help those who cannot help themselves; what I saw was a far cry from that. Why was it that I was so taken aback by these stories? It was the realization that although they were all cured of disease, they would never be able to escape the isolation. But their resilience inspired me. The woman was a victim of abandonment, but she found strength in independence. What I witnessed was the aftermath of disease at an unfamiliar scale. But this is not the first time I have seen a condition affect a person's life beyond physical well-being. Previous experiences I had in college had begun to shed light on the importance of holism in medicine.

This next paragraph continues the story of the first paragraph. We're now over 40% into the personal statement, and I'm not sure what I'm reading or why. I'm assuming this is a leper colony, but why was the student there? Why is the student asking themselves questions in the personal statement like, "Why was it that I was so taken aback?" What is the takeaway or the reason why the student is telling the reader this story? Here, it seems like it's only to say it's not the first time they had seen a patient before. We're also given a transition about college and the importance of holism in medicine. A lot of students will talk about realizing the "importance of XYZ in medicine," and my comment is pretty consistent: "You don't have to be a physician to realize the "importance of XYZ in medicine."

On entering college, I wanted to expose myself to the needs of my community through service. Every Thursday, when I visit the Hope Lodge, smells of freshly-baked cookies, friendly mingling, and familiar smiles welcome me. The atmosphere is lively as I walk in and greet residents fighting cancer, who often mention how they awaited my visit all day. I bring in a new craft or activity to do each week, which to them is an escape from the monotony of life. One typical day at the Hope Lodge, I decided to sit with a resident named Betty. She spoke of her passion for art and creativity, something she had abandoned on beginning treatment. I admired Betty's skill as a painter so I asked her to show me her techniques. I watched the contentment on Betty's face as she moved her brush intricately. It was then that I realized why I was there. My presence provided Betty an outlet to get back in touch with herself through art and companionship, in the face of illness.

The start of this paragraph is pretty cliché—trying to "sell" that the student is service-oriented. It doesn't tell the reader much. The student tries to tell a story of interacting with one of the patients through painting; however, there isn't a takeaway to tell the reader the importance of this experience for the student other than the student explaining that their presence was important for the patient. Instead, it should tell the reader why it strengthened their desire to become a physician. Ideally, the experience should be a little more focused on something around healthcare. While the experience doesn't have to take place in a more traditional healthcare setting like a hospital, it should still focus on healthcare. Playing bingo or cards with "patients" at a nursing home and telling the reader that made you want to be a physician doesn't really connect.

During the week, I also devote myself to service by tutoring at an after-school program for underprivileged children. I recall a day spending time with my tutee of 3 years, Haley, whose childish fervor for all things pink was unparalleled. Haley pulled me to a room to play princess while raving about her new sparkly pink necklace. However, the minute I pulled out flashcards, I found myself following her underneath a table. In that moment, I saw a piece of myself as a young child, terrified of failure. As a dyslexic, Haley struggled with her academics. I wanted to find a way to help her overcome her fears, so I spent months figuring out the best methods to help her learn. I discovered that I didn't need to separate work from play. I could lay out rows of pink sparkly beads on her desk, and demonstrate to her the concept of fractions. I could play dress-up with Haley and pretend we were princesses going to school and learning multiplication. It became clear to me that Haley learned best when her education was turned into something she loved doing. She taught me that teaching is more than conveying knowledge; it is about harnessing a person's personal experiences and strengths to diminish their weaknesses. This is how I see patient care. I am intrigued by the challenges a physician faces to bridge the gap between a patient's symptoms, their personal fears and values, and their experiences.

> *This is an example of a student trying to do too much with something that shouldn't be in the personal statement. The student is trying to use an activity to highlight what they learned: "Teaching is more than conveying knowledge." This takeaway doesn't scream, "I need to be a physician," but rather that the student thinks they know what teaching is about. The student then seems to force a connection to medicine, which I generally tell students to avoid in a personal statement. While the student does make a connection, they miss another opportunity to tell the reader why they want to be a physician, only that they are "intrigued by the challenges a physician faces."*

When I serve, I remember the woman in the purple sari, Betty, and Haley. Like them, every person has their own struggles inside and beyond their bodies. They remind me to uphold two things: the curiosity to hear a person's story and the compassion to help him or her overcome barriers. A career in medicine offers me a lifetime of opportunities to serve others in this manner while also healing them. Every experience has shaped my worldview and has solidified my decision to pursue medicine. When I started college, I wanted to be a doctor. Today, I understand what it means to be a rehabilitator, teacher, and a healer.

> *We have a repetitive conclusion for the beginning of this last paragraph. The student is mostly focused on serving and hopes that by showing they want to serve others, that this is enough to convince the reader they should be interviewed. A life of service is a noble life— but you don't have to be a physician to do it. There is nothing in this essay that tells the reader why they need to be a physician or even why they are interested in being one outside of being of service to others. The student then states they started college wanting to be a physician, but the reader doesn't know why they still want to pursue medicine.*

Personal Statement 2

My mind was full of stress as I stood on the starting block viewing the cold, clear water through my goggles. Diving into the water, I suddenly felt at peace, relaxed, and without worries as the only thing I heard was the water gliding along my body. As a varsity swimmer and student-athlete, I knew swimming was something I would enjoy for the rest of my life. However, my ability to continue swimming was doubtful when I was diagnosed with scoliosis. Swimming became a challenge as the curvature of my spine impacted my physical and emotional abilities. Every night and day, I wore a suffocating brace around my torso and became frustrated as I explained my diagnosis to people who stared at my back inquisitively. I thought I would have no hope of swimming again.

> *We start out with some good imagery of a swimmer on the starting blocks for a race and diving in to begin. We're then given a medical setback that impacted the student's life. This is one of the common seeds—it's not cliché, just common. The seed isn't wrapped up in a single paragraph, but I'm interested to keep reading, which is the goal.*

I remember the moment when my orthopedic surgeon said to me, "Tim, I need to surgically fuse metal rods to keep your spine straight." My heartbeat anxiously in my chest as my hand trembled. This all changed when my surgeon held my hand and explained how my condition could be cured through collaborative support from healthcare team members, allowing me to return to swimming. They showed me that it was possible to recover by empathizing, providing education, and treating me with a team effort even when I felt there was no hope. After my surgery, swimming was no longer difficult for me, and I was able to pursue my life-long interest, along with the peace it provided. I realized if medicine could have such a considerable impact on me, could it potentially impact others too? This question motivated me to start exploring a potential career in medicine. Little did I know that it would take years of exploration to find the answer.

Here, we have the rest of the student's seed. There is an interesting focus on collaboration, empathy, and education, which I worry the student is trying to highlight for some specific reasons, but at least at this point, they don't try to sell anything to the reader. This is a pretty good seed, although maybe a little long at over 33% of the personal statement.

I began volunteering at the Medical Center, accompanying patients to the surgery preparation room. I recall walking a patient who nervously told me about her surgery. As I securely held her hand, I felt it trembling and cold. Looking into her puffy eyes, I whispered, "I'm here for you." Instantly, her body language showed confidence and a smile appeared on her face. Once we reached the preparation room, she felt relaxed and her hands were no longer trembling. Although my gestures were seemingly simple, I provided her with a sense of security, comfort, and warmth that she desperately needed at the time. With the understanding that patients are still people and not just people with medical ailments, the responsibility of having purposeful connections with patients motivates me to become a physician.

This student does a good job of showing the reader their experience. The word choice helps paint a picture of what is happening—the student shows their empathy without actually saying they're empathetic. The student then has a good takeaway as to why this experience motivated them to be a physician.

In addition, I sought an opportunity to shadow Dr. S. In one specific interaction, I followed Dr. S as he sat in front of the patient and their family. "Jo," a young woman, spoke in a nervous and shaky voice about the lump forming on her breast. Considering how frightened she was, I was surprised to see the fear on her face replaced by a smile, which turned into laughter as Dr. S explained the treatment options. He was able to calm Jo through his charismatic and empathic demeanor and spoke in a clear way so that she completely understood that there was nothing to be afraid of. During post-op, I remember Jo telling him that she was able to fully pursue her own goals in life due to being cancer free. Dr. S has shown me the profound impact that physicians can make on patients through educating and comforting them. His sense of empathy and the impact he makes on patients has inspired me to become a physician.

This section focused a lot on empathy. The student did a good job in the previous paragraph to show their empathy without selling empathy. This time, the student is focused on the physician a little more than the patient and very heavily focused on empathy—possibly a little too much. The takeaway isn't specific to medicine. Seeing someone else being empathetic doesn't necessarily show the reader why you want to be a doctor.

To experience what it was like supporting and assessing patients, I became a clinic nurse volunteer. I clearly remember one of my patients, "John," a low-income elderly African American male who stumbled into my room. While measuring his blood pressure, I noticed his frail skin and limp body. He was ill and he told me that he had no motivation in life to see a primary care physician. The saddest part was every month he would come see me for his health assessment and tell me he had no loved ones or family to consent him for transfer to hospice. Even with the encouragement I gave him, he seemed to have given up life completely. As a student, I knew I did not possess the medical knowledge to treat him and it was disheartening for me to see someone in such a fragile state. Although this experience was not quite as gratifying for me, I felt I had the responsibility of his health as one of his only visitors. Even though it is inspiring to hear patients return to normal health, the story of patients like John are the ones that I hold onto, because these patients inspire me to become a physician and try again the next day.

This is an interesting story of direct interaction with a patient. These stories typically are the most impactful. However, I would recommend omitting the negative statement: "Although this experience was not quite as gratifying for me." Again, the takeaway could also be tweaked a little to be more specific to medicine. Trying again the next day isn't a physician-specific idea, so why the student is inspired to be a physician doesn't make as much sense. There is some good showing in this paragraph with an action word like "stumbled" and vivid descriptions like "frail skin and limp body."

Through my clinical experiences, I realized that physicians don't just heal patients long term, but impact them on an emotional level. I am drawn to becoming a physician because, uniquely among the caregiving professions, I can have meaningful connections to patients to provide them the treatment and guidance they need in their healing process. My highest goal is to practice medicine so that my patients can live their lives to their fullest, just as my surgeon did for me.

This is a good example of a conclusion that the student uses to talk about their goals and aspirations.

Personal Statement 3

The sun had begun to set as my family and I strolled through our backyard with my one-year-old sister. This was a moment of joy just before the trial that will forever be in my memory. Then it happened, as an eleven-year-old girl, I noticed that my baby sister was suddenly unhappy. I stood there holding my dear sister as my parents were alerted of the sudden change in her countenance. The incidences that followed were foggy and unreal; she was rushed to the emergency room. That same night, she passed away. The seriousness of her condition was known, and any moment could be her last, but her death remained a shock. Just a year before my sister was diagnosed with dilated cardiomyopathy. At the time of her birth, the doctors observed no abnormalities, but as months passed it was evident that something was horribly wrong. As a child, I witnessed the pain and suffering my sister experienced. The family trips to UCLA Medical Center became routine; I witnessed the physicians communicate with my parents the news of her condition. This experience as an adolescent awakened my first interest in medicine.

This is a perfect example of the very common "my family was ill/injured which led me to medicine." This is not cliché. This is their story. The student has to write about this to be truthful to their story and journey. It's a good opening. It could use a little more showing, *but besides that, I want to keep reading, which is what you want. The student could add a little more showing by writing about seeing their sister in the hospital—what was that like? What did they feel? What did they see?*

Another important point that I frequently discuss when giving students feedback on their essays has to do with the use of big words. It may seem smart to have the thesaurus open when you're writing your essay, but you should use very simple language as much as possible. The easier something is to read, the better. In the example above, I had to look up what "countenance" meant. It's not a normal word that one would hear in an everyday conversation.

As an eager yet unsure first-generation college student, I applied to my local university's pre-medicine track. Although being a first-generation student was difficult in various aspects, I pushed aside these obstacles and worked toward my goal to become a physician. As I navigated my undergraduate education, I was being prepared for future leadership opportunities. As a Sophomore, I became an Instructional Student Assistant and tutor for the Mathematics Department to assist incoming freshmen students who struggled with mathematics. The classroom setting encouraged social interactions with a diverse group, this helped me build positive interpersonal skills that aided in my subsequent interactions in a clinical setting. An obstacle that I overcame during my educational pursuits was providing monetary assistance for my two younger sibling's college education. I found that education is a journey dotted with sacrifice; but perseverance led me to strive towards my goal with fortitude.

The student diverges from "telling" their story to selling their story—being a first-generation college student and someone with interpersonal skills and connecting this to the clinical setting. The student also talks about financial struggles. I would probably consider this a red flag statement, and I would say it is too long. I would ask them why they wanted to share this with the reader. Are they showing what they have overcome on this journey? For the AMCAS application, the disadvantaged essay would be a good spot for this, as well as the discussion on being first-generation. For TMDSAS and AACOMAS, they could have included this here, but I would cut it down to something much smaller. The only tangible struggle mentioned was the financial struggle at the end. The rest of the paragraph about being first-generation doesn't belong in a personal statement. There are many variations of first-generation college students, and without further discussion in the disadvantaged essay, it doesn't tell the reader much. I think they could have said the following:

"There were many times during my college career when I questioned my ability to continue. Needing to financially support my siblings' college education forced me to work while taking

classes full-time. While challenging, I was glad I could contribute."
Those three short sentences are almost a 1/4 of the original paragraph, yet still show the reader obstacles they had to overcome.

Because of the unanswered questions regarding my sister's rare heart condition, I became intrigued by medical research. A lab position at my local university helped me understand how the methods of research operated. The complex interlays within research caused me to ponder how research related to medicine. I realized that medicine is constantly changing leading to the necessity for physicians to discover new cures and treatments. For instance, my mother was diagnosed at age thirty-one with glaucoma. The uncertainty regarding the cause of her condition and the absence of a cure for her rapidly progressing condition showed me that research plays a crucial role in the discovery and treatment of disease. Treatment of rare medical conditions as in my mother's case has become another motivation in my pursuit of medicine. In the future, I could provide a solution for the next generation who is experiencing the same conditions and uncertainties. Seeing the need for advanced medical care in cases such as glaucoma motivated me immensely.

Here, we have several examples of things I suggest students leave out of a personal statement. They are focused on research—this belongs in the activities section. They also have a few examples of generic statements, which don't help the reader understand the student. Here is one example:
"The uncertainty regarding the cause of her condition and the absence of a cure for her rapidly progressing condition showed me that research plays a crucial role in the discovery and treatment of disease."
Yes, research does place a crucial role in the discovery and treatment of disease. That doesn't tell me anything about the student or why they want to be a physician. In fact, it makes me wonder if the student should go into research instead of going to medical school. Remember that your goal is to show why you want to be a physician. This paragraph shows that the student likes science—"intrigued by medical research"—and that they want to use research to "provide

a solution for the next generation," which can be done without becoming a physician.

Following graduation, I was certain in my goal for medicine but the steps towards the goal were unclear. I realized the importance of patient care when both my grandparents were diagnosed with cancer. I was able to administer medication and provide emotional support for my grandparents during chemotherapy. I observed how patients are faced with the reality of death at the end of medical treatment. In these circumstances, I learned that a healthcare provider's duty is to be a positive influence for their patients. These events directed my interest in the clinical aspect of medicine. Another determining factor for my decision was the clinical experience gained as an urgent care medical assistant. A particularly impactful case as a medical assistant was when a patient was experiencing the symptoms of a myocardial infarction. During this occurrence all my focus was directed on the patient and of providing the best care to prevent further deterioration of life. My personal involvement in the communication with the physician and the medical staff was a powerful reminder of my desire to become a physician. The memory of my younger sister spending hours under the care of physicians and medical staff and watching both my grandparents take their last breath came to my mind. Being part of a medical team who shared the goal to administer quality patient care reaffirmed my aspirations in medicine. My task was small compared to the physician's, but I witnessed the physician effectively lead the medical team to the successful treatment of the patient.

This paragraph has a lot going on. I would recommend cutting this into a couple of smaller paragraphs with distinct purposes. The first part is talking about the student's grandparents. It's another example of talking about what they learned—"healthcare provider's duty is to be a positive influence." Remember, the goal is not to show what you have learned but to show why you want to be a physician. Also, for the purposes of your personal statement, be very specific about physicians and avoid using the generic term, "healthcare provider."

The second part of the paragraph starts to talk about a clinical experience in a very broad and generic way. I recommend being as specific as possible with each experience—tell the story of one interaction with one patient. Paint that picture. There is no takeaway that shows the reader why this was impactful other than that it reaffirmed their aspirations. I would follow-up with "Why?"

Working at various clinic locations, I witnessed the need for health education for the underserved populations. There were many individuals who did not understand how to prevent chronic diseases within their culture. I was convinced that the combination of medicine and public health was another beneficial approach to reach the minority populations who need educational tools to choose better lifestyle behaviors. Health education may have prevented many of the complications that my own family experienced. With this in mind, I became an intern for a program focusing on the prevention of type two diabetes among prediabetic patients. Witnessing how public health education and patient care can be combined led me to pursue my Master of Public Health. With a widened perspective, I hope to be better equipped as a physician to treat all demographics, populations, and cultures. Throughout my life every experience has prepared me to better serve a diverse world. A first-generation student with an undergraduate degree and soon to receive a graduate degree, with gratitude and desire I continue my pursuit of medicine. I believe that by becoming a physician, I will be able to inclusively serve society in my highest capacity.

Again, this is another long, multi-part paragraph I would recommend splitting into two paragraphs. The first part is mostly generic information—we need more health education, medicine, and public health resources to reach minority populations to help prevent complications. This is all true, yet it doesn't tell the reader much about the student. It's used here to give more résumé-type information, like the fact that the student obtained an MPH—a fact which would already be in their transcripts. After the MPH information, they do discuss their aspirations of wanting to treat all people and talk about their own experiences that will prepare them for that.

Personal Statement 4

Growing up in the countryside of Nigeria, my first memories of medicine were mixed with an overwhelming feeling of powerlessness. I was raised by my single mother, and our neighbors Ali and Umar became my role models at an early age. Lovingly, I called them "uncles." Unlike others in our modest neighborhood, these brothers were well-connected young professionals, and their success captivated me. Unfortunately, their lives were set for a tragic course. I was too young then to comprehend, but I now know that watching how AIDS corroded their lives, as they struggled for respect and survival, is what first compelled me to pursue a career in medicine.

> *We start off with our seed here. The student was exposed to the ramifications of AIDS at an early age. The student also shows that he is an immigrant with a very short mention of growing up in Nigeria. This may help some schools that are looking for that kind of diversity. It's not completely needed because your place of birth will be on the application. The only suggestion I would have for this paragraph is to do more* showing.

Ali first felt ill, and at our local hospital he heard, "you are dying from AIDS. There is nothing we can do." His disease progressed quickly, and dominated by shame and despair, he went into isolation aiming to hide the patchy dark spots on his skin, and his inevitable wasting body. Tragically, Ali died in an ambulance months later, as the hospital denied his admission. Umar would succumb to the same scorn of AIDS. Devastated by his recent loss, he desperately resorted to the dangers of black market medicine. However, the pills would soon prove futile in his fight, and Umar chose suicide over the suffering and social stigma associated with the disease.

> *We're given more backstory of the student's seed. This is the student trying to* show *more about what happened. It's still mostly* telling, *but he does a good job of letting the reader in on what he experienced.*

Decades later, openly identifying as a gay man, I sought the inclusion and acceptance I knew I could not find in our hometown. After immigrating to New York City, one of the epicenters of the HIV/AIDS epidemic, the effects of HIV disproportionately harming my community became even more concerning to me. As an active member of the LGBT community, I decided to join the fight against this virus. All along my uncles' history inspired me to learn and empower others affected by the condition.

> *Here we're given a little bit more about the student and his potential diversity that schools may seek out. What is important to see is that he's not saying it just to "sell" that he identifies as part of the LGBT community, but it connects to his path and exposure to medicine. This is a transition paragraph that really connects his experience growing up to the launch of his premed path.*

Driven by the desire to understand the human body and its pathologies, my initial steps into medicine began by resuming my undergraduate studies as a Medical Laboratory Sciences major. As I excelled in biomedical sciences, my early interest in infectious diseases granted me an internship at the NYC Public Health Laboratory. There I explored the diagnostic algorithms for HIV and other sexually transmitted infections and explored point-of-care testing through the NYC Sexual Health Clinics. I became greatly intrigued by the microbiological illnesses, and I wanted to translate the knowledge I learned in the testing centers into tangible help for patients in a clinical setting.

> *This is an interesting paragraph. It's starting to lead down a résumé path of what the student was doing all along the way. If you can read between the lines a little as well, it looks like the student is really talking about his love (and aptitude) of science—"desire to understand the human body" and "I excelled in biomedical sciences." The most important part of this paragraph, though, is the end: "I wanted to translate the knowledge… into tangible help for patients in a clinical setting." This is really the first time we're seeing the*

student's interest in clinical medicine. This paragraph is okay, and it may look similar to your story if you were interested in research before realizing you wanted a more clinical career.

I then became an HIV Testing Counselor at the Health Clinic (HC). My education there transformed into a tool able to impact the health disparities of not only the LGBT community, but also the immigrant communities. A couple, "Paulo" and "Mark" came in distress looking for professional testing following positive home tests. Paulo was frightened to seek help due to his fear to lose Mark, his only social support in the United States. We established a connection based on our similar backgrounds, and as I counseled and conducted Paulo's test, I was entrusted with his sexual and medical history in a time of vulnerability and anxiety. It was gratifying to use my biomedical knowledge to explain to the couple how the current state of antiretroviral treatment would allow not only Paulo to live a healthy life, but also minimize their concerns about a future serodiscordant relationship. My connection with clients at HC is thus far the most fulfilling experience in my career, and has only made me more eager to acquire the tools necessary to become a physician, the ultimate ally in the fight against AIDS.

In this paragraph, we are given a story of a specific patient encounter. Many students will write about an experience and talk broadly about all of the patients they helped. In contrast, this student does a good job of giving a specific example. He then goes on to talk about why it motivated him to continue down this path.

I began shadowing internal medicine and infectious diseases physicians so I could witness not only the rewards, but also the challenges involved in the care of these patients. Like the case of "Sonia," a frail AIDS patient who would not adhere to treatment due to selling her medication to support a drug addiction catalyzed by the social isolation experienced since her diagnosis. Sonia reminded me that infections carry implications beyond the ones caused by the pathogens. As infections sicken, they deprive the ill of human contact and regard, and this is where I feel I can make a difference. The task of applying medicine to fight stigma through knowledge, while reconnecting people through care, is the responsibility I was born for.

> *This story is one where the student is focusing on his interest, HIV/ AIDS, and the challenges for patients struggling with this condition. It could use more showing, but it does what it needs to do—shows the reader this student's passion—even ending with "the responsibility I was born for." That's a very powerful takeaway.*

I am dedicating my life to being a physician. I believe it is because I have seen and felt destruction, that I am so captivated by the hope that medicine can now provide for my clients. Because I remember what helplessness feels like, I believe in empowering patients through knowledge, compassion, and effective treatment. I understand medicine as a meaningful way of promoting health equity and, as a future physician, I envision learning and practicing within a healthcare team committed to creating transformative forces that work with, and as an advocate for, the patients. I plan to broaden my impact by seeking the tools to ease the suffering of not only those affected by HIV/AIDS but also all those affected by various health conditions. My goal is to treat each patient with the dignity and understanding they deserve, as I wish my uncles had been treated twenty years ago.

> *This is probably one of the best conclusions I have read. The student really highlights his aspirations, which support the rest of the focused story on HIV/AIDS. Do not worry if your story is not centered around a single topic like this—as long as you are taking the reader on your journey, as this student did, you will be doing what you need to do.*

Personal Statement 5

The opening chord of 'Here Comes the Sun', begins to fill the room. The faces of the audience change as they are transported through their memories to the moment the song became significant to them. Maybe it was playing during their first date or as their dad drove down a country road on the way to their family vacation. I look up from watching my fingers stroke the strings and a smile breaks out across my face as I see the joy that the music gives them.

> *This is an interesting opening, describing the student playing an instrument. It has some good showing, and I'm interested to learn more. Don't be afraid to highlight something like this if it's going to show your journey to medicine. Without knowing what the rest of the essay will discuss, my hope is that it leads to medicine.*

From a young age, the world has been my classroom since my parents chose to educate me at home. I spent my formative years going with my grandparents to the doctor because my mom was their primary caregiver. While other children were playing with dolls and pretending to be a teacher or mommy, I was taking temperatures and giving shots with my little medical kit that had a plastic stethoscope, reflex hammer, syringe, pen light, and blood pressure cuff. I treated my baby dolls, my mom, and anyone who would sit still for five minutes.

> *We're quickly off of music here, without any explanation why it was mentioned. Maybe we'll get back to music later. The student gives us their seed in this paragraph—being homeschooled and being around ill grandparents. The doctor kit description is a little cliché—hopefully, we'll get to some more specifics in the next paragraph. What is missing from this paragraph is the impact of going to the doctor's appointments. What did that mean to the student? How did it impact them or encourage them to explore medicine?*

Just after my fifteenth birthday, healthcare and medicine shifted from childhood play to everyday life. In October of 2010, both my mom and grandmother were admitted to the hospital. My mom had a section of her colon and her appendix removed because of diverticulitis, and my grandmother needed surgery to repair her broken hip. During this time, I researched my mom's and grandmother's conditions, the procedures they would have to undergo, and the types of doctors and medical providers that would interact with them. Through my research, I gained peace and an interest to study medicine.

> *Okay, so maybe this is the seed? The takeaway here is "I gained peace and an interest to study medicine." This contradicts the early discussion about playing with the doctor kit. My assumption as the reader is that they were interested in medicine long before this, but I guess the earlier discussion was just normal kid play.*

During college, I studied biology and chemistry, but the experiences that shaped me the most occurred outside the classroom. As a chaplain, I had the opportunity to utilize my experiences to comfort another person. A new freshman knocked at my door because she was missing home and wanted to watch NCIS with someone. As we watched the show, she started talking about home and her grandmother. Later, she disclosed the true reason why she had knocked on my door. Her mother had called to say they were taking her grandmother to the hospital, and my new friend did not want to be alone. Through our conversation, I realized that often all people need is to be heard, a quality that transitions perfectly to healthcare.

> *This is a good example of a student trying to highlight a skill they think the reader will be excited about. This experience isn't related to healthcare or being a physician—it's related to being a good listener. The student uses this story to show the reader they are someone who other people like to be around. They do not explain why they want to be a doctor, but they show why they think they'll be a good doctor.*

Through many different shadowing opportunities, I watched as physicians listened intently to their patients. I personally experienced not only the importance of listening, but also caring when I became the patient after a car accident. I can still remember how nervous and uncomfortable I felt as I sat waiting for my test results. My fears were calmed when the physician touched my knee and assured me that the results were good. Through his example, I knew that becoming a doctor is what I want to do as my professional contribution to society.

> *The example of being a good listener is carried forward to the student's shadowing experiences. Instead of giving a specific example of a shadowing experience, however, the student makes a quick change to talk about their own experience as a patient. I wonder why they brought up shadowing in the first place. The takeaway is, "I knew that becoming a doctor is what I want to do," but the student doesn't explain why. This is a very common mistake with takeaway sentences. This student is saying that it strengthened their desire to be a doctor, yet they don't let the reader know why it did. Why, when your fears were calmed, did that convince you that you need to be a doctor? You should always answer the "Why?" factor in your takeaway sentence.*

The hospital that I was admitted to after my car accident was closed a few years later, and I have watched the community change because of the closure. I realized how underserved my area was during a summer internship when I met two parents and their preemie twins. The closest children's hospital to the parent's community was 200 miles away. Thankfully, our local regional hospital had a NICU so the babies were able to be closer to mom and dad. I remember riding along with EMS to transport the twins to the hospital. My heart broke for the parents as I could not imagine what it would be like to be separated from children while they were so small and sick. My goal is to one day use my experiences and future education received as a medical student to serve the underserved as a physician.

> *The student focuses on a story of underserved patients to talk about their goal of helping the underserved. This is more focused on what the student wants to do as a physician and not why they want to be a doctor. You could potentially argue that serving the underserved is a "why," but you can serve the underserved in many ways outside of medicine as well. I'm always a little leery of these types of stories—is*

the student adding this in here to check off a hidden box for schools whose mission it is to serve the underserved?

The memory I described at the beginning was one of the many times I knew I was sharing my passion. A feeling that was more than surpassed when I held my first gallbladder. I will never forget the details of that day. Entering the operating room, I noticed the patient already draped, and the sterile field prepared for the cholecystectomy. As I was shown the best place to stand, the surgeon entered the room, and the procedure began. In the darkened room, lit by the glow of the monitor showing the inside of the patient's abdomen, the doctor began to isolate the gallbladder. My eyes were glued to the monitor in awe of the intricate details of the human body that I had only ever read about, but could now see.

The student ties back to their original story of shadowing in the operating room—sharing a passion. It's an interesting theme they carried forward. At this point, I'm not sure what they mean by sharing their passion and holding a gallbladder. Hopefully, we'll find out more in the next paragraph. You can definitely feel the excitement the student possesses. This is a very common focus for students—the excitement of shadowing or being in the operating room. I wouldn't focus on excitement—I want to make sure after 10 years, you still want to do this after the excitement has worn off.

As the surgeon removed the gallbladder from the patient, he instructed the scrub nurse to place the organ in a bowl and invited me to touch it. As I stood there holding the source of the patient's previous discomfort, I realized that the doctor had not just removed a diseased organ, but he had positively influenced the patient's quality of life. When I reflect on this day and how the actions of the doctor had a lasting effect on the patient's life, it affirms my desire to be a physician and I realize that I would do anything no matter the costs to do this every day.

After reading this last paragraph, I'm still left with the question of why they talked about sharing a passion. It doesn't really reappear.

We're left with a good takeaway, though—tying the doctor's influence on the patient to their desire to do the same. The final statement is a very common one—the student proclaiming they are ready for this, that nothing will stop them. Your goal isn't to convince the reader you're ready for this—since, truthfully, no one is really ready for medical school—but to show why you want to be a doctor and what you hope to accomplish. The accomplishment of that statement is missing in this conclusion. What does the student hope to accomplish as a physician? I'd be interested to know.

Personal Statement 6

Shakily standing up, my father steadied himself with his cane as he began his speech at my sister's wedding. "Not bad for someone who had their head cut open six weeks ago, am I right?" As the reception hall laughed and began to enjoy the rest of his toast, my immediate family graciously smiled, knowing our situation was not as light-hearted as put on. Diagnosed with metastatic melanoma, the months of May through September of 2004 had been full of neurosurgery, radiation treatments, and ultimately, grief for our family. While I was young and couldn't fully comprehend the situation, the physicians working on my father became close to my family and were an integral part in guiding us through the turmoil of our situation. The way that these physicians were able to inform and support my family through our cancer experience, advocate for my father when he desperately needed treatment, and offer themselves in service to helping my family was something that has since resonated with me, and originally implanted the thoughts of medicine into my brain. I wanted to be able to make that same kind of impact on other families going through similar situations, whether it be treating their loved one or be able to be there for them in their time of need.

We're given a good seed here, showing the student's exposure to healthcare because of their father's cancer. They also provide context about their age, which usually helps, so the reader can understand how long this has impacted their life. One thing to note is that your personal statement doesn't have to start with your seed. It seems to be the most common way students begin, but your story doesn't have to be in a specific timeline. As long as the reader can follow along, you can jump around.

As I continued growing up, medicine stayed in the back of my mind, however, I lacked confidence in my ability to pursue it. I focused on playing lacrosse and ultimately was recruited to play in college. However, my playing career was stopped abruptly due to an injury, I faced a new page in my life and began to focus on my academics. I had followed my advisor's recommendation to major in History and pursue law school. While finishing undergrad and working as a legal assistant, however, I found myself desiring more human interaction. I wanted the ability to physically help the people I was working with, work as a team with my colleagues, and have the knowledge and expertise to know I could directly impact someone's life for the better. As I began to look for a different career path, my father's doctors slowly crept back into my mind. I realized that medicine encompassed everything that I was searching for. Becoming a physician would give me the opportunity to continuously learn and expand my capabilities so that I can not only lead and assist efficiently as apart of a healthcare team, but that I would be able have the patient interaction and autonomy in decision-making I was yearning for.

This is a good detour paragraph with the student writing about why they didn't pursue medicine, even though they just explained to the reader why they wanted to be a doctor. My biggest concern with this paragraph—and you'll see it later as well—is that it looks like the student tries to define what it is to be a physician and then just lists the definition to convince the reader that this is what they are meant to be. The student lists human interaction, physically helping people, working as a team, knowledge, and expertise, which are also traits of most physical therapists, dentists, and other people in healthcare. They don't really explain why they are highlighting those characteristics, so my biggest question would be, why did they want those things?
Something else you might notice is the student tries really hard

to show the reader why they would choose to be a physician over any other healthcare career. They mention leading the healthcare team and autonomy in decision-making, which, again, a lot of students do in their personal statement; however, I don't think it's completely necessary. Yes, you need to understand why you want to be a doctor versus a nurse or a PA, but in your personal statement, you don't have to sell that. You should be prepared to talk about it in your interviews, though.

Continuing to take classes and gaining clinical experience, I began working as a dermatologic technician specializing in Mohs Micrographic Surgery. Like any typical day starting at seven a.m., I brought "Ms. Carter" back to our procedure room. She had developed two aggressive skin cancers on her nose that would likely take an extensive time to remove. As the day progressed, her tissue samples continued coming back positive for cancer cells, requiring further tissue removal. Going on ten hours in and out of the procedure room, I could tell she was feeling defeated. As I leaned her back into the chair, I knew nothing I said was going to make her feel better, but I did my best to cheer her up and to stay hopeful. I couldn't escape the feeling of helplessness and was upset in my limited role. I wanted to be able to do more for Ms. Carter than just try to cheer her up, I wanted to be able to have more responsibility and involve myself in a larger part of her care.

The student does a good job giving a specific patient interaction and showing the reader why it encouraged them to continue down this path. Since I wrote my personal statement book, I see the following statements more and more: "I wanted to be able to have more responsibility," or "I wanted to help in a bigger way." While this is the sentiment you want to get across, I don't think you need to specifically say it.

After nine stages of tissue removal, she was finally cancer-free and able to go home. As I ran to the waiting room and told her the good news, sweet 82-year old Ms. Carter jumped out of her chair absolutely elated.

This small paragraph doesn't show me any more of the student's journey, but it's nice to see happy endings.

Even with my smaller part of Ms. Carter's care, I left the room feeling like I truly made a difference. However, as I began to reflect on my experience with not only Ms. Carter but others as well, I realized that I wanted more out of those moments. Through a career in medicine, I would be able to obtain the skills necessary to combine human interaction and tangibly make an impact upon those in need, while also having the scientific propensity to make beneficial impacts in the development of healthcare for future generations. Working with people with a multitude of ailments has shown me that it can be an extremely taxing, yet fulfilling challenge. Through my experiences, I have come to understand that I will only be satisfied with having the full responsibility of a patient's care so that I can work to my maximal ability to help enhance their quality of life. While I remain on the journey of becoming a physician, I hope for the opportunity to attend medical school so that I can not only help cure and treat patients but also help guide my patients and community to further improve their health and raise recognition in the importance of disease prevention. As a physician, I plan to treat, educate, and be a patron for patients like my father, Ms. Carter, and others.

The student starts this ending paragraph with the "I wanted more" language I mentioned earlier, but this doesn't make sense here. The student tells the reader they want to be a physician, so obviously, they want more. This statement is more fitting for a nurse or a PA who realizes they want more. Make sure that what you're saying fits the rest of your story.

We are then taken back to the student making sure the reader knows they only want to be a doctor—"I will only be satisfied with having the full responsibility."

The last statement is a good example of what they hope to accomplish. I would have placed that separately as its own conclusion.

LETTERS OF RECOMMENDATION

*Note: Letters of Evaluation and Letters of Recommendation
are the same thing, and the name is interchangeable.*

Going through this process, relying on yourself is one thing; having to go through it and rely on someone else takes most premeds' stress levels to a new high. Combine that with asking others to "judge" you, and most students want to run away and hide. Yet, the letters of recommendation (LORs) that you need as part of your application are important—they help shed some light on who you are as an applicant.

The majority of the time, LORs are not going to hurt you. If someone is going to write you a bad LOR, they likely will just tell you they cannot write one for you.

LORs can definitely help you if your letter writer understands what they need to say to help give the Admissions Committee a glimpse into who you are. Let's dive into what an LOR is and what it is not.

What are Letters of Recommendation?

The LOR is not meant to be a sales pitch to the Admissions Committee on why you're the best student ever. It's not meant to turn your transcript into paragraph form—remember, the Admissions Committee has your transcripts. In fact, you don't *have* to get an LOR from only professors in whose classes you received great grades. If you made a connection with a professor in a class that you earned a C+ in, but that professor can show the Committee your work ethic, and how you overcame something in that semester to pull yourself up from an F to a C+, that letter will be infinitely better than a letter from a professor whose class you breezed by in with an A and who does not know you very well.

The first place where I point students when they ask what goes into an LOR is the AAMC resource *Guidelines for Writing a Letter of Evaluation for a Medical School Applicant*. This is good for professors and physicians, as well as new premed advisors, who might not know the components of a good letter.

Core Competencies

In the core competencies chapter, I gave you a rough idea of what medical schools may be looking for in an applicant. If your letter writer can incorporate some of these core competencies into their letter about you, it may make the letter stronger. When requesting a letter, you can give the letter writer the core competency information to reference.

Who to Ask for Letters of Recommendation

Most medical schools will have a list of the LORs they want from students. Unfortunately, this is a moving target and requires you to do your research into each school to determine what they want. Applying to a medical school only to find out that you're missing a required letter is a waste of time and money.

The standard requirement is to have LORs from two science professors and one non-science professor. Most students then also add in a physician with whom they have shadowed or worked. If you are a nontraditional student, review the school's website or contact the school directly to find out if they will accept a replacement evaluation from a work supervisor or someone else who may be able to write you a letter in place of a professor. Some of those replacement writers could include a volunteer coordinator, a supervisor at your job, a principal investigator, or someone else who knows you very well.

Most schools will give you a minimum and maximum number of LORs to send. I always recommend that students stick to the minimums. Admissions Committee members are busy. Make sure you are only sending letters that meet their requirements, and hopefully, these will be your best letters. More LORs could mean more opportunities for generic recommendations that don't help you.

Personal is Better than Prestige

A great letter of recommendation is not a letter from a world-renowned researcher unless that researcher knows you very well and can speak to who you are as a person. If you are only asking someone for a letter because of their status, please think twice. The best letters are from people who know you very well and can convey that in a well-written letter.

If you have maintained a great relationship with a community college science professor, a letter from this individual will be stronger than a letter written by a professor at a four-year university who barely knows you.

Physician Letters

Most schools do not require an LOR from a physician, but it is still standard for students to submit one. There is a myth that students can only apply to osteopathic medical schools if they have an LOR from an osteopathic physician. As of the writing of this book, only two schools, according to the Choose DO Explorer[6], state that they require an LOR from a DO—25 schools state they require either an MD or DO LOR.

It is okay to submit an LOR written by a DO to an MD medical school. It is also acceptable at most DO med schools to submit an MD LOR, though a DO letter may be preferred. If you are applying to any allopathic schools with a DO letter, make sure the letter written by the osteopathic physician is not specific to osteopathic medicine, or have them write you two letters, one to submit to

---

6   https://choosedo.org/

osteopathic schools through AACOMAS and one to submit to other (allopathic and osteopathic) schools through AMCAS or TMDSAS.

One of the biggest mistakes that students make is requesting an LOR from a physician they've only shadowed once; spending a few hours with a physician will not get you a strong LOR. The goal of an LOR is to show who you are, not just that you showed up and acted professionally. Hopefully, as you continue to shadow, you can have a conversation around having the physician write you an LOR. Let them know you are planning to ask for a strong letter of recommendation and see what the physician believes differentiates their strongest students from the rest. Following their recommendations may lead to a strong letter.

When and How to Ask for Letters of Recommendation

As a human being, you change over time. Every class, every semester, every year, you are growing, maturing, and adapting to your environment. An LOR from freshman year, more than two years before applying to medical school, will not capture who you are today. That doesn't mean you can't get an LOR from a professor from your freshman year. Many students maintain relationships with professors from earlier years and can still get very strong LORs from them.

Expectations are everything in life, and if you can start every new semester setting your expectations for the professor, they'll appreciate it, and it will result in better LORs for you. As soon as you can, I want you to talk to the professor with whom you have a relationship and from whom you will want a letter in the future. Set that expectation now. You can say something like this:

"Hi Professor Smith, I'm planning on applying to medical school in a couple of years. I've had a great experience in your class, and I would love to keep in contact with you so that when it comes time to apply to medical school, you can write me a strong letter of recommendation. Is it okay if I do that?"

After they say yes, don't ghost them. Continue to build that relationship with the professor—visit during office hours, help other students if you are not struggling yourself, and participate in class.

Remember, you are not asking for the LOR right then and there—you are setting the expectation that you might ask for one in the future. That way, when it comes to the end of the year, you have already had a conversation with the professor. They understand you are premed, they remember you from throughout the semester, and they are able to write a great letter because of the steps you took before the semester ended.

When you ask for permission to stay in contact, you are getting a loose agreement to communicate with that professor, and also an agreement for the professor to write you a strong letter of recommendation. If they decline, you will still have plenty of time to get another professor, and you won't waste your time with this one. There are obviously no guarantees here. The professor may not be at that school in a couple of years, and you might not be able to contact them, and that is okay. If the professor does change schools, and you can stay in contact, it's still okay to get an LOR from that person.

Start asking letter writers no later than February or March of the year you are planning on submitting your application. This gives the letter writer plenty of time to procrastinate and handle any other time commitments they have without feeling like they are letting you down. The last thing you want to happen is for a letter writer to be given short notice and then have them delay submitting your letter, which will ultimately delay your application. Remember, for most schools to consider your application complete, all letters you have assigned to that school will need to be submitted.

You may need to follow up with letter writers regularly to see if there are any issues. If you feel like your letter writer is not going to follow through, be aggressive in finding an alternative.

When Should Letters be Submitted?

Because you can submit your applications without your LORs, you do not need them at the start of the application process. Medical schools typically will not consider your application complete until the LORs have been sent to the school from the application service. The other parts of the application that are needed are your primary application, secondary applications, CASPer or AAMC SJT (for schools that require it), and your MCAT score.

As students aren't usually turning in secondary applications before mid-June, that is a good time to set as a strict deadline for you to have your letters. You should give your letter writers a deadline closer to the beginning of May to give you some flexibility if you need to scramble to get a letter.

A Strong Letter of Recommendation

When you ask your letter writer for a recommendation, you want to ask them for a **strong** letter of recommendation. You might say:

"Dr. Smith, as you may remember, I'm a premed student and applying to medical school next year. I had an amazing time in your class, and I was hoping that, based not only on my performance in class but also our conversations, communications, and what you've seen of me, that you will be able to write me a strong letter of recommendation."

If the professor says no, that's okay. If they say, "I use the same letter for every student," you can potentially still get that letter as a backup, or politely decline.

What if They Fall Through?

Sometimes, you will have a letter writer not be able to write you a letter. Whatever the reason, know that you should think through this scenario. It is fine to ask more letter writers than you need for a letter; if you do not need the extra letters when it comes time to submit your applications, you do not have to use them.

What if They Ask for a Draft?

Some of the people whom you ask for a letter of recommendation will ask you to write a draft, which they will then edit and sign. While this is a common practice, and there are plenty of templates available online if you search for them, I'd recommend trying to find another letter writer. If you must have a letter from one of these professors, do what you have to do in the end.

Do I Need to Finish My Personal Statement First?

Some students wait to ask for an LOR until they have finished their personal statement. I don't recommend doing this. Your letter writer *might* want to see your personal statement, or they might not. Don't delay asking because of an assumption. Even if you *know* they want a personal statement first, I would still ask before you complete your personal statement, so you are on their radar.

What Else Do I Need?

Very often, students come prepared with their personal statement, résumé, headshots, and much more when they ask for an LOR. Ask your potential letter writer(s) about writing you an LOR first, and then find out what they need.

Formally Requesting and Submitting Letters of Recommendation

Writing the LOR is one thing. Making sure it's signed, dated, and on letterhead can drive some letter writers bonkers. You need to ensure that your letter writer knows that all of these things are needed. Not every school may require these things, but many do; therefore, you should have every letter writer ensure that your letters are done in this way.

After they are written, the letters need to be uploaded into one of many places. Where your letters are uploaded and how the official communication is handled will depend on what service you use to handle your LORs. We'll go over the most common places next.

Directly to AMCAS, AACOMAS, and TMDSAS

Each of the application services has its own letter writer portals. If you want to go this route and you are applying to more than one application service, you'll have to create more than one request for each of your letter writers—one for each of the application services. The letter writers will then submit their letter to each service.

AMCAS

Go to the "Letters of Evaluation/Recommendation" tab and add a letter to be written. You'll need contact information for the letter writer, including their address and phone number. AMCAS will create a PDF that you can send to the letter writer to officially request the letter. Currently, AMCAS does not automatically email a request to the letter writer.

AACOMAS

Go to the "Evaluations" tab inside "Supporting Information" and create an evaluation request. You'll need the name and email address of the evaluator. You'll also request a due date and add a personal message to the evaluator. I would just add a short thank you here. Hopefully, you've already communicated your expectations with the letter writer. The personal message is just a small part of the full email; the letter writer will also receive directions on how to submit the letter.

TMDSAS

Click on "Letters of Evaluation" and add the letter writer's information. If you are using individual letters, TMDSAS has you fill out all letter requests at the same time before officially submitting them to be requested.

Interfolio

Interfolio is a popular service students use to store their letters and submit them to the application services when ready. The benefit of Interfolio is you don't have to wait until the application cycle opens up to start asking for letters to be written and submitted. Depending on your account level with Interfolio, the program can check your letter to make sure it is signed, that your name is spelled correctly, that the letter is on letterhead, and more.

TMDSAS and AMCAS both currently integrate with Interfolio. Interfolio can also get the letters to AACOMAS, but the process is a little different. After you create an Interfolio account, select "Request Letters of Recommendation," and then you can add your résumé, personal statement, and any other documents to Interfolio. Once you've finished your setup, click on "Request

Recommendation" and fill in the information requested. You'll have to add each new "Recommender." You can also add your personal documents like your personal statement to the request.

Whether you are using Interfolio, another service, or having your letter writers submit directly to the application services, you are not sending your letters directly to the medical schools where you are applying.

School Letter Service

Some pre-health offices have letter services for students applying to professional schools. The letter service is used to store your letters, similar to Interfolio. They will then send the letters to the application services. Check with your pre-health office to see if this is something they will do. If you're a nontraditional student, you may still have access to your school's letter service. One advantage of using your pre-health office's service is that they may review your letters and advise you on which ones to use.

Committee Letters

Some schools with pre-health offices will write what is known as a committee letter. Each office has its own policies and procedures, so check with your office as soon as possible to see if this is something you'll want to use. Many pre-health offices have very early deadlines for you to complete large parts of your application, so you may need to move your timelines up.

If your office does write a committee letter, you will likely need to send your individual letters directly to the committee. Check with your pre-health office about what they want—they may want your application materials and an interview with you before the committee will write a letter on your behalf.

If you have listened to my podcasts in the past, you know I'm not a fan of committee letters, as I don't see the point of them. Let's assume only 25% of undergrad institutions have them. Students applying from the other 75% of schools are still getting into medical school. Some medical schools I've talked to like the committee letter *if* the advisor has been at the undergraduate institution for a while, which gives the Admissions Committee a better sense of who the student is based on that specific advisor's writing.

My biggest issue with pre-health offices and committee letter policies is that many have minimum MCAT and GPA scores that you need to receive a committee letter. They are using your stats to determine if *their* time is worth it. I would argue that you are paying their salary with your tuition, therefore, they need to write you a letter regardless, but that is just not the case. Many of these advising offices track stats of who did or did not get into medical school. Obviously, the better their stats, the more they can advocate for continued funding from the university. Usually, they'll only track the stats of students receiving a letter from them.

Also, find out when the committee typically finishes and uploads the committee letter. A lot of pre-health offices become inundated with writing committee letters and don't submit them until later in the application cycle, which may hurt your chances of getting into medical school.

If your school offers a committee letter and you can't get one because they won't write you one, it likely will not hurt your overall chances of getting into medical school. You will need to submit letters individually, like most other students. You may need to justify why you are not using a committee letter; if that is the case, just be transparent with the process and why you decided not to use it.

If you are a reapplicant or a nontraditional student, find out if your pre-health office will still write you a committee letter.

Letter Packets

Some pre-health offices may not write a committee letter, but they will gather the individual letters and submit them together as a "letter packet." Unlike a committee letter, your advisor is not writing an evaluation to include with the letters. Letter packets are considered one letter in the application service and will usually satisfy all of the letter requirements a medical school may have.

Updating Letters as a Reapplicant

If you need to reapply to medical school, you should get new LORs. If you have LORs stored in Interfolio and you still want to use one of these letters, I would advise you to have the writer redate and reupload the letter. If they can improve their letter with updated information about you, that would be even better. Ideally, your letters are dated the same year as your current application. If you do need to ask for a redated letter, just send an email letting the letter writer know you had to reapply.

Adding Letters Through the Cycle

There may be a situation where you have the opportunity to get a letter from a new experience, or a letter writer who was supposed to get you a letter earlier on finally comes through, and you want to submit that letter to schools. In most situations, I would not send any extra letters to medical schools. Some schools may say it is okay to send an extra letter through the application service or as an update through their portal, but more is not always better. In almost all situations, I would go with what you have already submitted.

Double Letters for Certain Writers

One of my favorite tricks for the AMCAS application is that you can individually select which letters go to each school. If you have a letter writer who was formally on the Admissions Committee at Med School A, or at a minimum was an alumnus, you can ask them to write you two letters—one specifically for Med School A and another generic letter that you can send to every other school. You'll have to make sure when you are creating the letter requests in AMCAS that you keep them straight!

AACOMAS and TMDSAS do not allow you to pick and choose which letters you want to send to specific schools; they will send every letter to every school.

SCHOOL LIST

When applying to medical schools, there are a lot of options, with more seeming to open every year. With the ability to apply to all three application services, you theoretically could apply to every medical school in the country, over 170 of them. It's not feasible to apply to all of them, both for financial reasons and due to the time required to write all of the secondary essays. So, how are you supposed to choose where to apply?

Tiers of Medical Schools

Before I go any further, let me first remove the notion that there are tiers of medical schools. You've likely been made to believe that there are different tiers of medical schools by the undergraduate admissions process and premed forums. Unlike undergraduate institutions where the name of the school can unlock opportunities, graduating from *any* medical school in the US will allow you to practice medicine anywhere in the country

I'm not saying there are not great medical schools out there. Harvard, Stanford, WashU, and UCSF are amazing schools that boast tremendous stats and research dollars, and all of them are very selective. That doesn't mean **you** can't be just as successful as one of their graduates by going to your state medical school.

A lot of the top institutions are so caught up in their rankings that they continually seek out the students with the best stats, thinking that is what is going to make the school great. A lot of students with the best stats apply to the top schools to get the "best" education. Both of these assumptions are wrong, but they continue the cycle.

Instead of focusing on the name and the "rank" of the school, focus on the environment of the school and what you need to succeed.

Even with the change of USMLE® Step 1 going to Pass/Fail from a scored exam (Google it if you aren't sure what I'm talking about), you should not seek out the "top tier" medical schools only because you think that is how you will get the best residency. I recorded an episode of *The Premed Years* talking about the USMLE change. You can listen to that at premedyears.com/379.

Don't go to a "great school." Go to a school that will make **you** great.

Now that that is out of my system, let's dive into how students create school lists.

Building a List

Unfortunately, the most common way premeds build a school list is the complete opposite of how I recommend doing it. I hope that when you are done reading this chapter, you will be less likely to use this typical method to build your school list.

Stats

The majority of students will look at the Medical School Admissions Requirements site provided by the AAMC and apply to the medical schools whose "average" MCAT and GPA ranges match their own. They'll apply to those schools without much thought into other aspects of the school that may or may not fit them as a student, which is a huge mistake.

The first mistake students make with this method is misinterpreting the data the MSAR provides. The MSAR provides **median** MCAT and **median** GPA, not average or mean stats. Many times, a student with a science GPA (sGPA) of

3.6 will not apply to a school with a **median** sGPA of 3.8. The median number you see means that 50% of the class is above that number, and 50% of the class is below that number. Does a median sGPA of 3.8 predict a student with a 3.6 sGPA won't get in? Absolutely not.

The MSAR also provides the 10th to 90th percentile and 25th to 75th percentile ranges, which give you a better idea of the range of MCAT scores and GPAs generally accepted by that school. Even if you're below the 10th percentile number, you could be part of the 10% of students at or below that number. If you are a great fit for the school, let them tell you no *after* you apply—do not say no for them.

I hope that schools, the AAMC, and others will eventually put out the full data set of their accepted students to show the highest and lowest MCAT score and GPA of the students they have accepted or will accept in the future. Increasing transparency around the medical school application has always been my goal, and it needs to start at the institutional level. They are only hurting themselves, and students who would make great ambassadors of their school do not apply.

There are many other variables that go into an interview invite and ultimately an acceptance. MCAT scores and GPA play a big part of that, and students should be given the most amount of data possible to make the most informed decision possible.

Let's look at an example scenario. If the median MCAT of School A is 510 and you have a 507, does that mean you shouldn't apply to that school? Absolutely not. That means that 50% of the class is below that number—and so are you. If School A's 10th percentile number is 508, does that mean you shouldn't apply? Absolutely not. Here's the most important part: If School A is a school you would love to attend—a school whose mission matches yours, and you would be ecstatic if you received that phone call congratulating you on being part of their next class—then apply, and if it's not a fit for School A, let them tell you no.

The same logic plays out with median GPA. If the median GPA is a 3.7 and you have a 3.5, that doesn't mean you shouldn't apply to that school, nor does it mean you are not a competitive applicant at that school. All it means is your GPA is below the median for the data they provided to the AAMC for the MSAR.

You have to remember that MCAT and GPA are just two factors in your application. Yes, they are very important factors, and yes, they are needed to get to a certain point in the application process before someone reviews your application, but they are just two of many data points in the complete application.

Do not let historical data tell you no! The past does not predict the future, especially since your application is unique and has never been seen before— because it is **yours**.

I understand the cost of the application and secondary fees add up, and the cost of adding another school may be more than you're willing to pay, but I truly believe you are wasting more of your money by only applying to schools that "fit" your MCAT and GPA versus applying to schools that "fit" **you**.

Trends vs. Final Stats

Something you cannot see when looking at the MSAR, or any of the data from AACOMAS or TMDSAS, is what trends make up the stats.

If you finished school with two years of a 4.0 GPA, does that look better than another student with a 3.5 GPA every year, even if you both have the same exact final GPA? If you stumbled out of the gate in undergrad but picked yourself up and crushed your last couple of years, you're going to have an easier time overcoming a lower GPA. You can't see the stories of students when looking at the GPA and MCAT ranges in the MSAR. Those stories make a difference in an application.

If you *have* to use the MSAR to choose your schools, please look at the percentile ranges. The MSAR gives you the 25th to 75th percentile ranges as well as the 10th to 90th percentile ranges. Look at the 10th percentile; it means 90% of the class is above that number, while 10% of the class is below that number. If you are at or above that number, I would consider you a good enough applicant for that school. If you are below the 10th percentile number, then you are starting to get into a territory where you might not be competitive enough. The students in that range likely had other variables in their application that helped them overcome weaker stats. Maybe you do as well.

If you really want to go to a school whose 10th percentile number is above yours, it does not mean you shouldn't, or can't, apply. Go for it. Just understand it will be harder for you to earn an acceptance at that school. If you are below the 10th percentile for *every* school and you do not have a strong upward trend to show you have the academic ability to do well in medical school, then you might want to reconsider applying this cycle and possibly take more classes to strengthen your academic scores.

MD vs. DO

Before jumping into my thoughts on choosing schools, I want to talk about how to decide if you should apply to MD schools only, DO schools only, or both.

My general recommendation for most students is to apply to both MD and DO schools. With the increased numbers of students applying to all medical schools, increasing your chances of getting into **any** medical school is important. With so many variables in the application process, you do not know what may resonate with some Admissions Committees versus others.

There are very good reasons for only applying to MD schools. First, students who are thinking about doing a lot of work outside of the US may find that having an MD degree will cause fewer headaches when applying for a medical license in another country. The American Osteopathic Association (AOA) is working on getting full medical licensing privileges in more countries all the time, so hopefully, this will be less of an issue moving forward.

Second, while the negative DO bias is all but gone, there is still a strong-hold at some of the most competitive (and prestigious) residency programs. If you are a student who is looking to go into the **most** competitive fields, like Neurosurgery or Plastic Surgery, you may find that your application and connections need to be more competitive than an MD applicant if you went to a DO school. Don't get me wrong, as a DO, you can practice **any** specialty, and there are amazing DO Neurosurgeons and Plastic Surgeons out in practice right now.

The far majority of residency program directors I speak with on my podcast, Specialty Stories (specialtystories.com), state that they look at MD and DO applicants exactly the same and even state that some of their best residents have been DOs.

As I'm writing this, we are at the beginning of a new era in residency accreditation with a single GME accreditation system (do a quick Google search if you have not heard of this). It will be a few years until we see the impact of this change for DO students.

One this to keep in mind when applying to DO schools is that many have very large deposits if you are accepted. In many cases, the deposits are non-refundable (if you do go to the school, the deposits are generally put towards your tuition). It's a practice I want to see changed to be made similar to the regulations MD schools have from the AAMC. Unfortunately, the AOA has yet to take any action towards improving this practice. This has the potential of handcuffing you to one school, as you might not have the funds to pay another deposit if you get accepted later on at a higher choice school.

You can (and should) use my Application Cost Estimator at appexpenses. com to help with your financial decisions.

DO vs. MD Stats

Before I close out this section on MD versus DO, I need to bring up stats for MD matriculants and DO matriculants.

You'll see later on in the chapters about GPA and MCAT that DO stats tend to be lower than MD stats. This **does not** mean that DO students are worse than MD students.

There are many variables at play. The first of which is a self-perpetuating prophecy from premeds who are accepted to both MD and DO schools choosing to go to MD schools because they believe they will have more opportunities in their careers.

The second is what osteopathic schools have historically valued in their applicants. Osteopathic schools have always valued the nontraditional student, those who walked a different path to medical school. Prior to 2018, if you retook a class, AACOMAS would replace your old grade with your new grade. This favored students who struggled early but hit their academic strides later. It favored students who were lost and didn't know what they wanted, and when they finally figured it out, they flourished.

Yield Protection

Osteopathic schools know that students who have a 517 MCAT score (assuming they told their story well in the rest of their application—more on that later) are likely going to do well and get into their top-choice schools, and because of the students' own biases would turn down an invitation (or not even apply) to DO schools. DO schools may not invite that student, continuing the trend in lower stats. This is something called yield protection. According to Wikipedia, the definition of yield protection is when an "academic institution rejects or wait-lists highly qualified students on the grounds that such students are bound to be accepted by more prestigious universities or programs."

There are many reasons a MD program will not interview a highly-qualified student. Students from a state like Texas may not get an out-of-state school interview because the Admissions Committee may have data showing that even if they accept that student, the student is likely to stay in Texas because of their ties to the state and very low tuition. Other schools that have a very specific mission may not interview students they don't believe will ultimately fit that mission.

At the end of the day, the stats for DO matriculants are heavily affected by the students who keep applying based on those historical stats and the false premed narrative around MD schools being *better than* DO schools. It is just false.

My Recommendation for School Choice

My recommendation goes against the common premed philosophies on choosing schools. My recommendation is to pick schools based on where you want to go to school (which part of the country, what type of weather, proximity to family, proximity to friends, etc.), curriculum, class size, and many other smaller factors we'll talk about below. Look at schools in the areas you want to be, and do some research into those schools as you think about applying there. You need to pay close attention to the mission of the school and see if your story fits with their philosophy.

Let's dive deeper into some of these variables.

Curriculum

What sort of curriculum do they have? Is it a traditional curriculum, where they teach all the subjects separately (anatomy, physiology, pharmacology, etc.), or do they teach a systems-based curriculum where they teach the cardiovascular system, including the anatomy of the cardiovascular system, the physiology of the cardiovascular system, the pharmacology of the cardiovascular system, etc.?

I went to New York Medical College, which, at the time, had a traditional curriculum. Having gone through it and knowing the different systems now, I think I would have done much better in school and been much more engaged in the first couple of years if I had been in a systems-based curriculum. You have to understand your learning style. You have to understand the way you like to absorb information to see which curriculum may be best for you. Many schools are moving towards problem-based learning, while others are approaching a flipped classroom. I'm not going to dive into all of the nuances and definitions of those curricula here, but know there are a lot of differences and you should do some research as part of your list building.

These are all different types of learning environments that you may or may not succeed in. You have to understand who you are to determine if that school may be a good fit for you. Some schools, like Lake Erie College of Osteopathic Medicine, in Erie, Pennsylvania, offer different tracks of learning for students. At the University of Colorado, where I have been on faculty, we have a lot of problem-based learning. Many students like it; some students don't. Either way, if it's required by the school and you choose to go there, then you are stuck with that program, so dig into the curriculum and make sure you are setting yourself up for success.

If the school you want to go to, based on location or another reason, does not have a curriculum in which you think you will thrive, that is okay. It means you may need to work a little harder to succeed—it doesn't mean you will fail.

Class Size

Class size is also important to many students. Can you picture yourself in a small class of less than 100, or would you feel more comfortable in a class of 300? I always think about one student who was really excited about applying and getting into one of the largest med schools in the country because they were interested in the different types of students with whom they could connect. They were interested in all of the different personalities, interests, and diversity. You may prefer a more intimate learning environment with a much smaller class size.

Culture

It's hard to understand what the culture of a medical school is by reading a website or looking at the MSAR® (Medical School Admissions Requirements™). You ideally should visit the school, so try not to immediately limit yourself with your school list. Before the school visit, keep your mind open; do not have hard lines drawn in the sand when it comes to what school is your favorite or not. I have talked to many students who attend an interview or an open house and realize the school they never gave any thought to might actually be their top choice. After visiting a school, considering the community of students and the facilities, and after talking to the administration and faculty, what was at the bottom of the list might now be at the top.

You won't know until you're actually on campus, so keep an open mind as you go through the process and try to go to as many open houses as you can. When you are on the interview trail, ask questions, explore the area, talk to as many students as possible, and hopefully, you'll end up at the school that best fits you.

Summer school tours are very common for high school students exploring universities, but for medical schools, it isn't the same. Some medical schools hold open houses, so check in with a school you may want to visit for their available opportunities. I do not recommend showing up unannounced.

Mission

To try to get inside the heads of the Admissions Committee, look at the school's mission statement. The Admissions Committee is trying to build a cohort of students whom they think will best meet their mission. Let's look at the University of California, Riverside's current mission statement:

The mission of the UCR School of Medicine is to improve the health of the people of California and, especially, to serve Inland Southern California by training a diverse workforce of physicians and by developing innovative research and health care delivery programs that will improve the health of the medically underserved in the region and become models to be emulated throughout the state and nation.[7]

If you are from San Francisco and have shown no experiences working with a population similar to Inland Southern California, or you are from outside of California with no strong ties to the area, then you likely will not even get an interview, even with great stats, because you are not the student they want to train. Going to a school whose mission does not fit yours may lead to an increased risk of burnout or other obstacles on your journey to the career you have envisioned for yourself. They are doing you a favor by making sure you are not where you don't belong.

Out-of-state versus In-state

When applying to medical schools, one thing to note is where your state residency lies. Public medical schools are funded by the state and typically have some sort of mandate for the number or percentage of students they can accept from in-state versus out-of-state. Let's look at Texas, for example. Texas law states that public medical schools can only accept *up to* 10% of their class from outside of Texas.

If you are applying to public schools in a state outside of your state of residency, review their stats to see how friendly they are to out-of-state applicants. Texas, for instance, with the law mentioned previously, is not very "out-of-state friendly." Some schools, in contrast, like the University of Michigan, which is a public medical school in Michigan, historically accepts 50%, or more, of their class from out-of-state.

As you are building your list, look at the schools, including public schools outside of the state, to see if you should apply. One thing that will help as you're

---

7   https://medschool.ucr.edu/missiondiversity

building your list of out-of-state public schools is whether or not you have what I call "significant ties" to that state.

For instance, back when I applied to medical school as a Florida resident, my family had moved to Colorado. I applied to the University of Colorado School of Medicine, which is a public school, and I was an out-of-state applicant. I didn't have the best stats (roughly equivalent to a 502 MCAT), but I still received an interview. I was able to tell the story of my visiting family in Colorado for years and wanting to end up there as well. In the secondary applications, a lot of the schools will ask: *If you are not a resident, why are you applying to our school?* You'll have the opportunity, just as I did, to discuss your ties to the state and why you are interested in going to that school.

For students who are in a state without a medical school, do some research into any nearby states with medical schools to see if they are *friendly* to residents from your state more than other states. The University of Washington School of Medicine's WWAMI Regional Medical Education Program was created specifically for that purpose. WWAMI is an acronym created by the states it serves (Washington, Wyoming, Alaska, Montana, and Idaho). It was established in 1971 to help students applying from those Western states without medical schools to get the medical education they need and, hopefully, return to their home state to serve their population.

Private Schools

While there are a few exceptions, most private schools do not have a preference for in-state versus out-of-state students. Private school tuition is generally much higher than public schools, especially public, in-state tuition. Public schools generally receive funding from the state, which covers a portion of each in-state student's tuition. This is why their out-of-state tuition is much higher and more in line with private school tuition.

International Students

If you are an international student, obviously, all medical schools are "out-of-state." Getting into a US medical school as an international student is hard but possible. I've done several interviews with international students who have been accepted into US medical schools, discussing their journeys. You can hear those at premedyears.com/371 and premedyears.com/341.

Building a school list as an international student is harder and requires you to dig into each school's entry in the MSAR. If they say they accept international applicants, look at how many international students apply, how many are interviewed, and how many are ultimately accepted or matriculate. If a med school states they accept international students, but the actual data doesn't show it, you are probably better to move to the next school. You will need to do a lot of research to see which schools are the friendliest to international applicants.

There are two big concerns for medical schools accepting international students. The first is the fact that international applicants cannot receive federal loans to pay for medical school. Applicants will have to prove they can afford some or all of the cost of tuition, depending on the medical school. Some medical schools may have a large enough "bank account" to give loans, or even full scholarships, to international applicants they really want at their school. Let's hope you are one of those students!

The other concern is obtaining a work visa after medical school. If you are accepted and graduate but then have visa issues and cannot start your residency program on time, or at all, that might give the medical school a bad reputation or cause accreditation concerns.

Understand that as an international applicant, you can attend a US medical school; however, there are more barriers in place and less wiggle-room for mistakes. Despite that, with the right amount of effort and determination, it is possible.

Do your homework and look at all the schools where you're thinking about applying. Ensure you're not wasting any time or money applying to a school that will likely not accept you solely based on your residency status.

Acceptance Rates

A lot of students will try to gamify the application process and look at each school's specific acceptance rates. This doesn't actually work. There are a lot of students applying to each medical school, and acceptance rates range anywhere from about 2% to 4%. That doesn't mean that *you* only have a 2% chance of getting into medical school. Remember, on average, the acceptance rate for all students applying is closer to 50% when considering every student and each of the application services.

With many medical schools still having prerequisite courses, required letters of recommendation, or other nuances in their application process, many students applying likely haven't met those requirements. When you also consider in-state versus out-of-state residency, as noted earlier, many students are applying to schools where they have close to a zero percent chance of getting an acceptance, making the numbers look much worse.

The bottom line is to avoid looking at acceptance rates for each medical school when building your list.

Tuition

The very last thing I want you to look at is tuition. Too many students put tuition higher up in priority, limiting where they are applying, such that they don't get accepted in their first cycle. Not applying to a school that is $20,000 more expensive per year ($80,000 over the course of four years) and delaying a year of earning potentially $160,000 or more doesn't make mathematical sense. Before you limit yourself based on tuition alone, make sure you are looking at the big picture. If you have multiple acceptances to medical schools, and you have determined that every school will be an amazing fit for you, that is the time to look at the tuition of each of the schools to determine which one is going to be the least expensive to attend.

School List Size

Unfortunately, as the number of students applying each year rises, so does the number of schools each student is applying to as well. According to the AAMC, in Table A-1[8], on average, students applied to 17 medical schools in the 2020-2021 cycle. When I first started looking at this data several years ago, it was around 14 schools.

---

8   https://www.aamc.org/system/files/2020-10/2020_FACTS_Table_A-1.pdf

For DO applicants, on average, each student applied to almost nine medical schools [9].

I don't recommend applying to more than 25 schools. If you have great stats, activities that demonstrate why you want to be a physician, and a solid story that will show an Admissions Committee why you're doing this, you likely don't need to apply to more than 15 schools, especially if you've properly researched each school's mission to find those that will fit you well.

Applying to medical school is expensive, and each school that you include in your list will increase the cost. Again, check out appexpenses.com for my free application cost estimator.

Even if you have unlimited funds, don't apply to too many schools. You will burn out from all of the essay writing that comes with each additional secondary application you have to complete.

Should I Delay My Application?

Before starting and submitting your application, you should review the things you've done to ensure you are ready. In the flying world, we call this the go-no-go decision. Do you have the experiences, stats, mindset, support, and finances to continue with the application? Or should you take a step back and wait another year? It's always the question that thousands of premed students ask themselves every year as they work on their application. About half of the students who start an application every year don't actually complete it [10]—including students who are actually planning on applying that year and students who are researching what the application looks like for a subsequent year.

If you are in a situation where you are questioning whether or not you should submit, maybe you should listen to your gut. There is a difference between being nervous about the outcome and doubting if what you have done is enough. Delaying your application because you are not satisfied with your clinical experience giving you enough exposure to formulate why you want to be a physician is different than delaying it because you don't think you're good

---

9   https://www.aacom.org/docs/default-source/data-and-trends/2019-aacomas-applicant-pool-profile-summary-report.pdf
10   https://news.aamc.org/medical-education/article/7-things-know-about-amcas/

enough. Having concrete reasons why you are questioning your application differs from imposter syndrome.

I know that sounds confusing, so let's work through some examples. If you think your grades are borderline, then take some time and register for more classes to show an upward trend. If you think your grades are borderline, but you push forward with your application, and you don't get into medical school, in hindsight, then it is easy to say you should have waited. The question is, where do you draw that line?

If you think your MCAT score is close to or below average, it's almost never the wrong decision to delay your application to do some more intensive MCAT prep, get a higher score, and apply the following cycle. If your clinical experience, shadowing, or research hours are low, and you're not comfortable with your position, the safest and most financially prudent decision is to delay your application.

With the competitiveness of the medical school application process, you really need to apply with the best application you can put together, not something you are rushing because of pressure from your family, or because you think you are getting too old, or any other reason.

Playing this game is a lot of armchair quarterbacking, where hindsight is 20/20. If you apply and you're rejected, you might say, "Well, I knew I probably shouldn't have applied, but I did anyway." I don't want you to get completely wrapped up in this game because it is an impossible game to play.

My general stance in these situations is to be conservative. If there are aspects of your application that are questionable, I will almost always recommend delaying an application to fix or improve those issues and then applying with a stronger application. The application process is draining. It's expensive. It is traumatizing when you don't get in. What I typically recommend is to apply one time with the strongest application possible.

The Go-No-Go Checklist

Let's think about the different parts of the application. I want you to look at certain aspects critically and decide if they might be issues for the Admissions

Committee. This is almost exactly the same exercise you will have to do if you don't get into medical school to see what might have gone wrong.

On this side of the application process, we're being more proactive, on offense, trying to see if we can fix anything now or if we're going to have to delay the application. If you're reading this book six months or more before you apply, you may be able to fix some of these things, so you don't have to delay your application.

MCAT Score

I know you're tired of hearing about the MCAT, but it is a big factor in the application process. Once you get past MCAT score minimums, the rest of your application kicks in, and you can get to the holistic admissions process. You need your MCAT score to get you to that point, though.

When you are in the middle of your semester, and you are working to support yourself, trying to do research and prepare the primary application, your MCAT prep is usually something that starts to slip.

If you are starting to worry about your MCAT prep, instead of stressing out, I would recommend pushing it back until the end of the year or the beginning of next year. Tell yourself, "You know what, I'm going to take a gap year. It's okay. I need to relax a little bit." I don't want you to burn yourself out over the application process because you think you *have* to apply this year.

The same thing goes if you are retaking the MCAT, and your prep isn't going well, and you think you need to push back your MCAT test date into July or August. Anything past June for an MCAT test date, in my mind, is starting to push into being "late." Students always message me after I post something about the end of June, and they ask, "What about mid-July?" Last time I checked, mid-July is later than June. Will you be okay? Maybe. Will it hurt a little more because you are later in the cycle? Maybe.

The later you push back your MCAT test date, the more I will tell you to stop pushing it back by a week or a month and just wait until the next calendar year to apply. Again, take your time, work on the rest of your application, and move forward.

GPA

If you haven't yet, go to Mappd.com and sign up for a free two-week trial and enter all of your courses to look at your GPA calculations and trends. If you have a downward trend, a stumble coming into the finish line of your undergraduate career, you may want to consider delaying your application and taking more classes for another semester or two to prove to the medical schools that the stumble was just a fluke.

If you are below a 3.0 cumulative and/or science GPA, you may want to raise your grades to get them above a 3.0 with postbaccalaureate classes or a master's degree.

Clinical Experience

Lack of clinical experience is unforgivable when you are applying to medical school. You have to prove to yourself that this is what you want to do and what you like. To do that, you need clinical experience—you need to put yourself around patients.

If you are looking at your application, and you don't have a lot of recent clinical experience or a lot of clinical experience in general, then I would work on it immediately or delay your application.

This is one of the biggest things I see with students when I talk to them at the beginning of the application cycle. I will ask about their MCAT and GPA scores, as well as their shadowing and clinical experience, among other information. If they say they haven't had any significant clinical experience, recently or at all, I will immediately tell them they should stop the application process to get clinical experience, and then apply next year. If it is early enough in the application cycle and they already have some hours, but it has been a while, I will tell them to get back into it as soon as possible, and they might still be able to apply this cycle.

Sometimes that can save an application. Remember, though, the Admissions Committees aren't dumb, and they can see something added to your activities list at the last minute. If it looks like you are trying to check off a box, they are not going to like it.

Unlike shadowing, where you should be with physicians, you can count time in different types of clinical settings as clinical experience. For example, if you are spending time in a podiatry office and interacting with patients, you can count that as clinical experience. However, I would suggest that any clinical experience outside of the more traditional settings not be the majority of the clinical experience that you have.

Try to get at least 100 hours of clinical experience—obviously, the more, the better, assuming consistency as well.

Shadowing

Lack of shadowing, like lack of clinical experience, can be a red flag. Even if you are coming from a healthcare-related field, like nursing, you need some shadowing experience to see what that physician does outside of your interaction. If you have a ton of scribe experience and very little shadowing, many medical schools will consider that scribe experience to be good enough.

Shadowing should be done with an attending physician if you are going to count it in your hours. Attending physicians are those who are out of training—not in residency or fellowship. You should not count shadowing a PA, chiropractor, physical therapist, podiatrist, or any other healthcare provider or area of healthcare in your activity list; you need to shadow attending physicians. Many schools also want your shadowing to be in the US

Try to get at least 50 hours of shadowing with consistent hours throughout the application year. Consistent hours will show you're not just checking off a box. Consistency doesn't mean 20 hours a week; it could mean five hours a month.

Research

Research is probably the most confusing part of the medical school application. Is it required? Is it not? How much do I need? Do I need to publish or present a poster for it to count?

If you are at this stage evaluating your application, and you have zero research experience, that is okay. You can get into medical school without any research. There may be a few schools with strict requirements, but even research-heavy schools like UCSF have told me they look for students without research experience as well.

If you have other experiences that show you are interested in diving deep into subjects, whether related to school or not, that helps. Research doesn't even have to be related to medicine. If you're an engineering student who did research on bridge designs, that will suffice. Recently, I had a student who was changing careers after being a geology professor, and her rock research was a big part of her application.

You don't have to publish or present a poster for any of your research to be included on your application. Schools understand that being able to publish a paper is something that comes with a lot of luck. You need to have joined the project at the right time to have contributed something valuable enough to be included on the paper and to have made any conclusions. A paper has to be submitted, reviewed, and accepted, and often that takes time as well.

Some students think they have done "research" when in actuality, it was data entry. Make sure that if you are going to include research on your application, you understand what was being studied. If all you are able to talk about is how you entered data into the computer's software, not only will that not look very good, but it most likely will not be considered research.

When students ask me if they should go out and try to get involved in research, my suggestion is always to try it out. See if you can find a physician doing some clinical research and volunteer as a research assistant. Find a lab doing something you are interested in or ask your professors if you can participate in any of their research projects. Try it, and if you don't like it, that is okay.

Dual-Degree MD(DO)/PhD Programs

If you are applying to MD(DO)/PhD programs, then the conversation around research is completely different. A lot of students apply to dual-degree PhD programs because they like that they are free with a stipend. The National Institutes of Health funds many programs through the Medical Scientist Training Program. Be warned: free medical school is not a reason to apply to these programs.

Dual-degree PhD programs are looking for students with extensive research experience who can join their programs and continue the research at their institutions. If you don't have sustained, robust research and you are unsure of your future as a physician-scientist, you probably should not apply to these programs.

Time

If you feel like you are running out of time for everything, whether that is MCAT prep, writing your personal statement or extracurriculars, or fitting in last-minute activities, the last thing I want you to do is to get frazzled and have your grades and/or your MCAT prep start to slip.

Recovering from poor grades at the end of your academic career can be challenging, time-consuming, and expensive. Retaking the MCAT is dreadful, and if delaying your application means you can focus more on your classes and your MCAT prep, then I want you to do that and delay your application.

Many premed students now are purposefully taking gap years, pushing off the MCAT until after they graduate, so they don't have to take classes while also preparing for the MCAT. This is a very strategic tactic that reduces stress and ensures the student is focusing on each part of the process independently. This might be something you want to think about.

At the end of the day, the application process is long. There are a lot of moving parts, responsibilities, and necessary steps. If you feel like any part of it is beginning to slip, and you're feeling burned out, it is okay to say, "I'm not going to apply this year."

Delaying your career for a year, starting your career at 30, and working for 30 years, versus starting it at 31 and working until you're 61 isn't anything in the grand scheme of things. Take care of yourself now. If you can make the application work for this cycle, great; if not, remember that delaying your application is not a failure, but a strategy for being better prepared.

EVERYTHING AFTER THE PRIMARY APPLICATION

SECONDARY APPLICATIONS

One of the unique things about the medical school admissions process is the fact there are several parts to it. It is always interesting to see the reaction when students first hear about the whole application process, or the look on parents' faces when you tell them their child needs more money for "another" application.

What are Secondary Applications?

The secondary application process begins after you submit your primary application to the centralized application service. Secondary applications are generally a set of essays that each medical school wants you to write. Because each medical school has a particular mission, they want to ensure every student they are going to interview and ultimately accept will fit that mission. Secondary applications allow the medical school to ask very pointed and specific questions to help them determine if you are going to be a good fit for their class, their community, and their mission.

Not every medical school uses the opportunity to ask specific questions, and you may find that the questions asked are pretty generic. You should still use this opportunity to answer the essay prompts to the best of your ability and, after doing a lot of research into the school, try to express how you fit the school's mission.

Part of the secondary application process also involves money. Each medical school charges a fee (set by each school) in order to submit your secondary essay.

Some schools do not have essays and only use one-way video interviews or situational judgment tests like CASPer or the AAMC SJT.

Are Applications Screened Before Sending a Secondary Application?

After you submit your primary application, most schools will automatically send you secondary applications. Most schools do not look at your GPA or MCAT when deciding whether or not they will send you a secondary application. They are **not** looking to see if you are a qualified applicant prior to giving you that secondary application.

The application process is a long, tedious process that involves a lot of resources for the Admissions Committee at each medical school. Screening primary applications takes time and even more resources. Not screening before sending a secondary application is a way to help cut down on the resources, and time, required to get through the application cycle.

It is up to you, as the student, to understand if you are a qualified *enough* applicant. If you are applying to Harvard with a 2.4 GPA and a 490 MCAT, you are not likely going to get in no matter who you are, so that is probably a wasted application. One of the hardest parts of the application process is choosing medical schools where you have a decent chance of getting an interview. I always say you have a 0% chance of getting in if you don't apply and more than a 0% chance if you do apply. That doesn't help, though, when you are looking at minimizing the number of applications to schools.

This is one part of the process where I wish medical schools were more transparent—what is the lowest MCAT and GPA they would ever consider? It's hard to look at the median or average stats to see where you might fit in. If schools gave a little more data, it would help you a lot. You can, however, call each school and see what their cutoffs are if they don't publish them. Some will give you those numbers while other schools will not. It doesn't hurt to ask, though. Maybe if enough students ask, they will start publishing the data.

Unfortunately, it's not in the best interest of the medical schools or the AAMC to be more transparent. The more students who apply, the more money that they receive in application fees.

When Will I Receive Secondary Applications?

Medical schools don't receive the first batch of applications for a little while after students can first submit. For osteopathic schools, that date is historically mid-June. For allopathic schools, it has historically been late June. Remember that you can typically submit your AACOMAS applications immediately after they open. You have to wait until the end of May or the beginning of June before you can submit to AMCAS. Starting in 2021, TMDSAS also has a delay between when the application opens and when you can submit it.

That means, even if you submitted your AACOMAS application on May 16th and were verified on May 20th, your application won't get to medical schools until mid-June. That's when you can start expecting notifications in your email inbox about requests to complete a secondary application.

If you are applying later, after the first wave of applications, you'll likely get those secondary requests shortly after you submitted your application—even before you're verified by the application service.

One of the benefits of submitting your primary application early is the downtime between submitting and when secondary applications are actually requested. This is the perfect time to start pre-writing your secondaries. I'll have more info on that later on in this chapter.

Common Secondary Application Essay Prompts

Because medical schools are looking for students who "fit" their programs, many of the essay prompts will revolve around who you are and what you will add to the class. Some very common prompts will ask why you are interested in that specific school, how you fit with their mission, what diversity you bring, etc.

Other very common essay prompts revolve around your journey. The prompts may ask you to write about obstacles, breaks in education, and any other parts of your application you want the Admissions Committee to know about. You can see common secondary application prompts, example responses, and feedback later on in this chapter.

Compared to the personal statement, I think secondary application essays are much easier to write. You are typically answering a very specific question instead of an open-ended prompt like, "Why do you want to be a doctor?" As long as you are answering the question with a good writing style, i.e., expressing your story by showing instead of telling, then you should be fine with your secondary essays.

Alternative Secondary Applications

Some medical schools are moving away from essay prompts for their secondary applications. CASPer and the AAMC SJT are newer tools that many medical schools are using as part of their secondary application process. We will cover them in the next chapter.

AAMC's VITA, the CASPer Snapshot, and other one-way (meaning you are not talking to anyone; your webcam is just recording you for viewing at a later date by the medical school) video interview tools are also gaining traction. These video interview tools are asking very similar questions to the common written essay questions in the secondary applications.

Secondary Application Turnaround Time

One of the biggest mistakes students make with secondary applications is waiting to write the essays until they actually get the request from each medical school. Students may think the schools will only send them a secondary essay if they are qualified enough to receive one; therefore, they wait to see if they get one before they start writing the essays. As we talked about already, the majority of schools will automatically send you a secondary essay, so you need to be prepared for the tidal wave of essay prompts coming your way.

You should, to the best of your ability, prewrite the essays for each school's secondary application. Most schools do not change their essay prompts from year to year, so you can find the previous year's prompts at secondaryapps.com and start working on them for your application cycle.

If one of the essays changes, or even if all the essays change, that is okay. The essays you are writing will likely be useful for other schools' secondary applications as well. After you finish five to ten secondary applications, each additional one starts to become repetitive. The work you are putting in for the initial essay prompts will help you as you move forward writing more essays.

Ideally, you want to turn around secondary essays within two weeks of receiving them. Some medical schools have actual deadlines for secondary applications, but most do not. Pay very close attention to everything coming in, and prioritize the ones with deadlines. I have seen some schools with 5- and 10-day secondary deadlines.

If you are able to prewrite your secondaries, then you can turn them around much more quickly than that. If you don't prewrite your secondary essays and you've applied to 15 MD schools, then as soon as your application is submitted to the medical schools, you will likely get 15 secondary application requests very, very quickly. You will then need to scramble and write 30 to 45, if not more, essays and turn them around very quickly.

It is in your best interest to prewrite your secondary essays in order to turn them around as fast as possible without getting overwhelmed. Every year I talk to students who stop applying to medical schools because they become completely overwhelmed with the secondary essay process and don't turn in their secondary applications to medical schools.

Remember, because of rolling admissions, the sooner your secondary application is submitted, the sooner your application can be considered complete and reviewed by the medical schools.

AACOMAS and TMDSAS Specifics

AACOMAS has the ability for medical schools to have students submit secondary essays from within the primary AACOMAS application when designating the school. Each school has to sign up to be a part of this, and so far, it's not very popular, so I don't know how long it will continue. If a school you are applying to through AACOMAS has its secondary prompts in AACOMAS, you have to go to a designated website to pay for the secondary application fee. You do not pay for it through AACOMAS.

TMDSAS currently has one school, Texas A&M University College of Medicine, that requires you to create an account in a special portal to receive a secondary. Unlike every school that will send you an email, you must be proactive with their secondary.

Examples

Below are examples of essay prompts and real responses from students with my feedback.

We have all tried something and failed. Describe a situation, or an experience, you've had when you were unsuccessful. Tell us what you learned from this experience.

My first year at Duke I was failing both Calculus and Organic Chemistry at the same time. My academic skill-set in high school had failed to prepare me for the rigors of a pre-health science major in an extremely competitive university. I knew drastic changes had to be taken or else two failing grades would result in academic suspension for a semester, so I visited the academic resource center and set up personal appointments with both instructors to discuss my options. I made the decision to withdraw from the course in which I had the smallest chance of recuperating the failing grade and focus all my academic attention, with the help of a tutor, on the remaining final exam. The experience showed me how to stay grounded while analyzing a situation in which there seems to be no good option, but the most important thing it taught me moving forward academically is to put aside the fear of being stereotyped or succumbing to the belief that I was not smart enough to belong and seek help.

Typically, when asked about failure, it is ideal to use non-academic failures. This student took a different route, and that's okay, as this prompt doesn't specifically say to avoid academic examples. Based on this prompt, the student does a good job of writing about what happened, why they think it happened, and what they are doing to work on these shortcomings. Based on the prompt, they have answered the question and hopefully eased any concerns about their academic abilities. I recommend staying away from academic (including the MCAT) failures in secondaries and in the interview because failing inside a classroom is common, and the story behind that usually doesn't lead to a better understanding of who you are as a student. Telling a story of failing as a leader in an activity or job will reveal more about you.

Much of health care delivery involves teamwork. In what endeavor have you engaged that required a team approach? What was your role and what did you learn from working with this team?

Managing a product development team requires constant team communication and coordination. With almost a dozen people working on one product across multiple states, it is easy for small misunderstandings to snowball into radically differing opinions on which direction to go when refining the product's design. By periodically providing updates and keeping short-term objectives in line with the long-term goal, over the last three months we have taken an idea of something that I believed first responders needed in the field and evolved it into a tangible proof-of-concept poster to be presented to potential investors. Much of the company's success has come from seeking mentorship from more experienced entrepreneurs and listening to peers willing to contribute words of advice and warning from their personal experiences. This opportunity has opened my eyes to an entirely new way that health professionals with field-specific knowledge can work together to make a difference in patients' lives.

You'll see from how this student responded that they didn't really answer the prompt. By being generic about what was going on and not talking specifically about their role, they avoided the questions. While the reader can extrapolate some of the answers, you should be more direct. For example, the prompt asks, "In what endeavor have you engaged that required a team approach?" It also asks for the student's role. This student should have been more straightforward and stated:

"As the product manager for a 12-person product development team, I was responsible for..." Instead, the student was not specific and tried to sell their skills by stating: *"Managing a product development team requires constant team communication."* Does the student know that because they were the manager or because they saw the manager doing this? Make sure you're specifically answering the questions without giving generic responses.

Give an example of how you made a difference in someone's life and explain what this experience taught you about yourself.

Mac has been my best friend since we played football together at the age of seven. The year Mac re-accustomed to civilian life from the Marines was especially difficult as he ended an eight-year relationship, suffered his fourth concussion, relapsed into drug dealing, and lost Marine brothers to suicide. That summer, our candid conversations reinforced in me the profound cascading effect that words can have and grounded my perspective. We talked about how far we had come since childhood and I emphasized how quickly all that could be taken away if he continued dealing drugs. I listened to his fears surrounding his mental and physical health and answered every question I could, promising I would research the ones I could not answer. I showed him that he could be honest with his physician about his side effects from medications and discuss alternative treatments like CBT. I left my hometown knowing that Mac was in a better place and that because of this, I myself was in a better place.

The first thing I noticed from this answer is that it seems to be missing a response to the second part of the question "...and explain what this experience taught you about yourself." The other thing concerning me about this response is it's focused on healthcare. Whenever I see a response focused on healthcare for a prompt that doesn't discuss healthcare, I worry that the student is trying to force a narrative of "Look at me, I can do 'doctor' things." I think this is a good example of making a difference in someone's life, but if there was another story of a non-healthcare-related experience, I would likely have chosen that one. This example also "tells" a little too much and doesn't "show" us enough.

What motivates you to apply to our school?

I stumbled into global health in my first semester of undergrad because an introductory course filled the time-slot left by a class that I had switched out of. I had never heard of global health before then. I quickly discovered that global health occupied the intersection of my passions for improving quality of life, approaching problems from a macro perspective, and a desire to return to the Latin American region to serve the underserved. The MD/MPH program would be the continuation of my academic and professional endeavors in global health dating back to 2013 as a research assistant doing data entry of field surveys. The school's involvement in Latin American countries through international electives demonstrates to me as an aspiring physician and cultural anthropologist that community involvement and cultural competence are prioritized in their education of future physicians. I am motivated because this school has just the tools to help me become the physician that I dream of being one day.

At first glance, you might think this is a well-written essay answering, "Why this school?" In truth, the response is too generic. The student writes about an interest in global health and the school's MD/ MPH program, which is generic. The one extra piece of information provided is about Latin America. One can assume the student is from Latin America because they state, "return to Latin America." That piece of information specifically helps this one school understand their motivation since a lot of schools have MD/MPH programs. The last sentence is broad since any medical school will have the tools to help you be the physician you want to be. You want to be as explicit as possible when talking about why you're interested in a medical school.

Choose one of the following areas in which you have interest. Comment on how you would hope to impact medicine in this area. Please do not exceed 1500 characters (about 250 words).

Biological and Biomedical Sciences

Underserved Populations

Entrepreneurial Medicine

Other (specify)

Underserved Populations

I have experienced firsthand the negative impact that residing in a medically underserved area can have on a population. While living, volunteering, and shadowing in these places, both in the US and internationally, I have developed a passion and interest to help those without the means to obtain adequate healthcare. I have a strong desire to someday provide care in an underserved area as a physician as a result of these past experiences. Growing up in multiple small towns, I have learned how close-knit the communities are and how they often function as one cohesive unit. These are the types of towns that raised me to be who I am today. They celebrate their successes together and mourn their losses together. I have experienced both the successes and losses that deeply affect entire communities like these. The health of these individuals is no less important than the health of others, yet it is more difficult for them to receive healthcare because of where they live. While volunteering on mission trips to Guatemala, I have seen this impact to a greater extent, where many of the patients we saw had never received healthcare in their lives and were facing many chronic health problems. I want to give back to the type of rural and underserved communities that raised me by providing healthcare to them as a physician, and to be a part of the glue that holds that community together.

It seems like this student has a lot of specific experiences that would tie in well with serving the underserved, but unfortunately, they were very generic with how they explained their experiences. Saying "growing up in multiple small towns" and "I have experienced firsthand the negative impact that residing in a medically underserved area can have" are as specific as this student gets when "showing" the Admissions Committee what it was like to be a part of the underserved community. This answer would be much better with a specific story recalling what they saw growing up in this underserved area. As much as you can, pull in anecdotes from your life to answer the questions; this helps the reader understand who you are much more powerfully than when you just give general information.

At the State University Medical School, we are committed to building a superb educational community with students of diverse talents, experiences, opinions, and backgrounds. What would you as an individual bring to our medical school community? Do not exceed 1500 characters (about 250 words).

I have had a passion for leadership that has strengthened with age and experience. Over time, I have worked to develop my leadership skills so I can help my peers to the best of my ability. While leading multiple organizations on campus, I always try to remember a few key qualities that have made many of the people I look up to great leaders. Communication skills has been one of the leadership qualities I have worked on the most. Being able to inspire and persuade my peers while effectively providing them with as much information as I can has been a key constituent in my leadership development. Empathy is an important component of leadership that I have learned while serving both in leadership and clinical roles. Talking with many pre-health students about the struggles they face has taught me about the importance of understanding the feelings of another to be able to provide them with advice they will take to heart. Although not always easy, taking ownership of mistakes is a quality that every leader should embody. I have no shortage of past mistakes, and as a role model for pre-health students I have been open about these poor decisions, talking about what I've learned from them to help my peers learn from them as well. This has been very important in my leadership development because of the honesty required to build trust with others. I have been able to develop these qualities to enhance my leadership ability and have also carried them over into other facets of life.

Similar to previous essays, the student doesn't specifically answer the question of what they would bring to the medical school community. The student begins the answer with, "I have had a passion for leadership that has strengthened with age and experience." Does that mean the passion they have for leadership is what they'll bring, or the leadership itself? Like a good politician, the student then turns the question around to make sure they answer it the way they want to by listing all of the qualities they wanted the Admissions Committee to know they had. Remember to respond with specific answers to specific questions. If the question is, "What are you going to bring?" and it seems in this essay it is leadership, then give the reader a particular example highlighting your leadership skills. Then show how you think that leadership (or whatever skill/trait/experience you're going to bring) will add to the community.

What experience have you had that has given you insight into the patients you hope to eventually serve? (1500 char)

I grew up in multiple rural communities, and wherever we lived there was a substantial amount of underserved people, whether it be food, housing, or healthcare. Most places that we lived we had to drive at least 30 minutes to the nearest urgent care or to see a provider or any kind, and even then it was usually hard to get in to see them because they had to serve such a broad area. My interest for helping the underserved medical population began while I was still in high school, witnessing its prevalence in multiple different hometowns. Now that I work at a hospital in a smaller city I am still exposed to this underserved population because of the long distance they must travel to be seen here, due to the fact that there aren't enough physicians for them to be seen in one of the smaller towns closer to them. Seeing this deterrent to a patient's ability to receive the best and most convenient healthcare for them has been both frustrating and motivating for me. It has been frustrating in the sense that this problem is so common across the US and serves as a barrier to the patient's health and well-being. It has motivated me to combine my passion for healthcare, knowledge, and leadership to dedicate my service to these populations as a physician. Although it is still very early on in the process, I know that I want to give back to the types of communities that raised me to be who I am today by addressing that shortage in physicians.

> *This student does a very good job of providing a specific example to show the reader where they are from. "We had to drive at least 30 minutes to the nearest urgent care or to see a provider of any kind" helps paint a picture of the challenges this student endured just to see a doctor. From there, the student can write about their interests, and the reader understands the student's past, which gives a framework and legitimacy to the response.*

What will be your greatest challenge in becoming a physician? (1500 char)

My biggest challenge in becoming a physician falls outside the realm of the classroom or hospital. My family is, and always has been, important to me and will continue to be a large part of my life no matter what the future holds. My ability to balance my time between school, or work, and my family will be crucial to my success as a medical student and eventually physician. Although I am currently a busy college student, I am only a few hours away from home and can easily make the trip back on some weekends to see my family. However, this is a luxury I will not likely have going forward and I fully expect to encounter some bumps and bruises in finding some solution where I am still able to keep in relatively close contact with them, and acclimate to that change. Another aspect of that balance also includes finding some time to relax for myself and time to exercise. I have not had trouble so far with the balances between these areas of life, however I am preparing for the commitment to school being far larger going forward, requiring me to be more strategic in these balances, and the potential for multiple sacrifices to be made. I am willing and ready to make the necessary sacrifices, so long as I am able to maintain a healthy harmony between these facets of life in order to achieve my dream of working as a physician.

> *This is a good answer for the prompt, as the student highlights what they think will be their biggest struggle. That said, while I think this answer is okay, there is the potential for the reader to be concerned.*

The very last sentence, "I am willing and ready to make the necessary sacrifices, so long as I am able to maintain a healthy harmony," tells me that the student isn't willing to do what is necessary if they can't maintain that balance. I would prefer the student to finish with a stronger message, conveying that no matter what, they will make the necessary sacrifices.

Discuss a time in your life that demonstrated your resilience. (1500 char)

When I came to college I was dating a girl I had gone to high school with. We had been good friends since I moved to that high school, and I had become a close friend of her entire family too. My girlfriend's mom had been diagnosed with cancer multiple times before we had been dating, but she had fought it off each time. Our senior year of high school she was once again diagnosed with cancer, however this time it was much more aggressive. With her parents being split up, my girlfriend and I were often charged with taking care her younger siblings. Seeing the impact their mom's health had on them was truly devastating, even more so the fact that this wasn't the first time. I still vividly remember the silence while driving them all to the hospital to visit their mom. We both attended the same college, and when we left I could tell that she was having a very hard time being away from her family in a time like this, so I did my best to be there for her. Her mom was in and out of the hospital through the year, until she passed away early sophomore year. Although I was saddened, I did my best to temporarily push that out of my head to help my girlfriend and her siblings in any way I could, with meals, groceries, and transportation because I could not imagine the amount of pain they were feeling. Although we're no longer dating, we're still great friends and I always make sure she knows to call me if her family ever needs anything, and I know her mom is still watching over me.

This answer doesn't seem to answer the prompt at all. If anything, it would be the girlfriend's family's resilience, not the student's, that is on display. I can't stress it enough—you have to make sure you're answering the prompt as specifically as possible.

Describe a time when you did not receive what you felt you deserved, and how you reacted. (1500 char)

The medical mission trip I am coordinating for this January has been an official campus organization for three years. One of the requirements of each campus organization is they must have a faculty advisor. The first coordinators who associated the trip with our campus were running low on time, and picked a professor they knew through research. That faculty advisor informed them that she would be fine with handling the bank statements, but outside of that she didn't know much about healthcare or the trip, outside of her being on our Premed Committee. A few years later she has continued her laissez-faire advising of the organization. Our other coordinator and I discussed the pros and cons of having her as an advisor, and decided that our club would benefit more as a whole from an advisor looking to get more involved in learning about the trip and perhaps providing some mentorship. We also wanted someone more involved in the healthcare profession, considering all volunteers on our trip are pre-health students. We talked to our current advisor about the situation and she actually said that she wasn't looking for this to be a long-term role for her, and she would be happy to pass the organization on to someone else, but would be willing to remain our advisor until we find someone. I feel that being open and honest in our conversation with our current advisor and her willingness to compromise with us will benefit all our organization's volunteers this year and for years to come.

The responses to this essay prompt are always fun to read. A lot of times, they are train wrecks. It is very hard to answer this prompt in a way that doesn't seem like you are complaining, which I would say is the main goal with this prompt. Let the reader understand what you think you deserved, offer some explanation of why you think you didn't get it, and then what you learned from it. This student does a decent job of explaining what they learned from it, but they seem to be complaining. Saying that the advisor had a laissez-faire attitude is judgmental and critical. Focus on the situation and on yourself, and don't attack another person.

Please describe a personal or professional challenge or conflict that you have experienced. How did you resolve it? What skills, resources and/or strategies did you employ? DO NOT write about the MCAT, a course, or an academic issue.

I was born with a permanently detached retina and have never had any sight in my left eye. Although this is definitely a characteristic that makes me unique, I live my life no differently than any of my normal-sighted friends. I do not have any driving restrictions, reading impairments, or problems otherwise. Many times the only way people can tell I am single-sighted are the cataracts and calcium deposits in the eye.

Like many children growing up, I did have to deal with bullying because I was different. We moved around the state multiple times for my dad's job, and at each school I met a new challenge with my eye. Depending on where I went and what age I was, some of my peers thought it was cool, some thought it was weird, and others honestly didn't even notice. A crucial part of my development was my acceptance of that abnormality and being willing to explain it to those whom asked. I have learned to make light of the situation and develop a sense of humor around the topic, because it can often make others more comfortable talking about it as well. At this point in time, there is nothing I can do to fix it, and I have come to treasure that part of me that truly does make me a unique person.

Although I may not have perfect depth perception, I did not allow this challenge to stop me from my love of sports. I played football, basketball and baseball all throughout my childhood, and became the first single-sighted varsity quarterback and point guard in my high school's history. I was never treated any differently than any of the other players and I was motivated to train to become the best player I could be during the season, and in the off-season, so that having one functioning eye would not even have the potential to be used as an excuse for poor play. My impaired depth perception taught me the importance of muscle memory for the way I played sports, and I ended up leading the basketball team in free throw percentage for two straight years. I honestly did not believe my vision problem to be detrimental to my ability to perform, but I was able to use it as motivation to train and perform at a high level. I was able to extend that motivation past the fields and courts, and into the classroom.

Being single sighted has not just taught me a great deal about myself; it has molded me into the person I am today. I have learned that although protective glasses or goggles may not have been considered cool while I was younger, they were, and continue to be, vital to my whole future. It has developed my ability to persevere and taught me that making excuses does not help when in pursuit of a specific goal. My single-sightedness has not been a deterrent for me, but a tool for growth and development.

This student did a great job articulating their experience as someone born with sight in only one eye. They painted a picture of what it was like to interact with others, function in life, and play sports, and how their condition shaped them. Bringing up disabilities in an application could bring in some unwanted bias, but this student was, hopefully, successful in easing any concerns about what they were able to do despite their differences.

Please state your reasons for applying to Private University School of Medicine. (2000 characters)

There are many reasons I'm motivated to be a medical student at the Private University School of Medicine. First and foremost, learning how to be a physician in the classrooms and clinics affiliated with such an excellent medical school would help me become a compassionate and knowledgeable physician. An aspect of the curriculum I feel to be unique is the lifestyle management course. Being in undergraduate, I can't yet understand the impact that becoming a medical student will have on my lifestyle, let alone when I someday become a physician. I like that the course provides opportunities for self-knowledge and growth as it addresses both the physical and mental stressors that being a physician will likely create. I feel the longitudinal clinic would give me the opportunity to apply some of the things learned in the classroom to the real world. That would help me retain information better and further enjoy learning the material. I would also really like to be a part of the Special Clinic. I have had experience seeing and serving underserved populations in rural areas and on medical mission trips, and I would like to continue this at Private University, potentially at the Special

Clinic. Another reason I'm motivated to go to Private University are my ties to the Midwest. I haven't experienced the type of genuine kindness that I have experienced in this region of the US elsewhere, and it's a factor in why I want to practice medicine here. My family is very important to me, all of whom are located in the Midwest. I feel that this school is just the perfect distance from home for me to further my education while still remaining fairly close to them. I have a couple friends who go to this school, and I have heard nothing but great things. They've shown me what they can do in their free time and talked to me about all the amenities the school provides. I would be extremely grateful for the opportunities to utilize all of these as a medical student at Private University.

Looking at this response, there is only one part of the answer that is specific to the school, which is when the student discusses the "Special Clinic." Even with that particular piece of information, a free clinic (which I'm assuming this is) to aid the underserved isn't very specific, yet many students use it when answering "why this school." The student's first response was to praise the school: "...such an excellent medical school would help me become a compassionate and knowledgeable physician." Every medical school will offer you the ability to become a compassionate and knowledgeable physician. Be careful with overly general responses and responses that are just there to show admiration for the school. It's okay to put the location in a response if it relates to having a support structure, but I would suggest placing this reason last on the list. Also, referencing the location and how nice the people are in the Midwest is not a strength of the school. Remember to focus on the school itself. A common mistake with this type of prompt is mentioning the hospital(s) affiliated with the school. I do not suggest this because the question is about the medical school, and the hospitals are not the medical school.

Given the distinctive educational philosophy and integrated curriculum at our school, describe how your personal characteristics and learning style would fit the institution. (200 words)

I tend to be a very organized person, so seeing the graphical breakdown of the four curricular elements through all three phases of medical school was very appealing to me. I learn the best when I am able to apply the things I am studying on paper to the real world, which is one reason I really enjoy science. The ability to work closely with physician mentors, opportunity for early clinical experiences, and the use of the simulation lab would allow me to better retain and enjoy the information learned in the classroom. I have also discovered that I am able to able to learn and perform better when working effectively in a group, whether being the leader or a following another's lead. Working closely with my fellow classmates outside of class, in clinical experiences, and in the Synthesis and Application Modules would help me to continue strengthening my communication and collaboration skills while effectively learning material that will help us all become excellent physicians. Coming from multiple rural communities, I value close relationships with others. The individualized design for medical students would provide me with an opportunity to build those same types of relationships in the big city.

The very beginning of this response probably wasn't needed, as their organizational skills have nothing to do with the prompt. In addition, liking science is definitely not needed here. The student finally gets into some specifics when mentioning the physician mentors, early clinical experience, and simulation lab. Remember that your job with these types of prompts isn't just to list the specifics of the school but to also reflect on your own experiences and how they relate to what you are listing. It would have been a nice bonus for the student to highlight the school's educational philosophy so they could then focus on their personal characteristics and learning style and how they fit with that philosophy.

Describe the steps you take to reduce your personal stress when confronted with difficult situations.

When confronted with a difficult situation I step back from the situation to whatever extent I am able, to remember the big picture. There's a reason behind each stressful situation, and in order to address that situation I first search for the root of the cause. Finding the source of the problem reduces a substantial amount of the stress because I know exactly why I feel that way and it allows me to start to formulate different potential solutions. Through much practice, I have become thorough when it comes to weighing the positives and negatives of each outcome. I will often make a list of pros and cons if time allows it, because another way to reduce my stress is to make sure I am picking a solution that I am confident with. Over the past couple years, I have been extremely lucky to build up an amazing web of support. When I am feeling stressed out I will often reach out to my family, friends or pray, to ask advice or just vent to them. Their encouragement has extinguished so much stress and has acted as a launch pad to help me overcome difficult situations.

> *While this response does answer the question and tells the reader what this student does in difficult situations, it would have been much better to give an anecdote to highlight a specific instance in which the student used one of these techniques to reduce stress.*

Reflect on a time in which you personally gained more from an experience than what was expected. (1000 characters)

For a field-experience class I was required to volunteer for a certain number of hours, and I choose to help out with an adult fitness program. I expected to assist with exercise classes, to give participants workout plans, and to spot them to ensure safe exercise. I gained those skills and so much more. I have developed some very close relationships with many of the participants. We know all about each other's families, pasts, fears, and dreams and we will sometimes meet up outside of the program just to talk. While helping these people achieve their fitness goals, they have given me so much advice. They've taught me that are some lessons that are hard to learn unless someone with that exact experience tells you about their experiences, and I have taken so many of their tips to heart. I owe each of them a huge thanks because I could not have overcome my mistakes to apply to medical school without their support and encouragement, and I will definitely remain in touch with them.

> *Similar to the previous prompt and essay, this response answers the prompt, but it could be much better with an anecdote of an interaction with one of the student's close participants. This would show the reader what the student felt and experienced with that relationship.*

What do you hope to gain from your Medical College experience that will make you a better/different physician? (1000 characters)

At Medical College, I hope to utilize all of the physician faculty to absorb all the information that I possibly can. I want to build relationships with them to potentially learn from them outside of the classroom as well as within, and carry those relationships past my time in medical school. I plan to volunteer in the Community Service Initiatives Program to help out the west side community, continue my passion for service, and continue to develop and strengthen my sensitivity and genuine kindness to those in need. Coming from multiple tight-knit rural communities, I value building strong relationships and the relationship that I would be able to foster with a physician-mentor through the school would give me many excellent tools to develop my knowledge and clinical experience. The interprofessional approach of Medical College would also give me a more comprehensive view of all that goes into patient care and allow me to understand the jobs of everyone I work with, directly and indirectly.

> *Hopefully, by now, you can see what I see with this response. This is a pretty generic response to the core question, "Why this medical school?" Being able to "utilize all of the physician faculty" is something this student can do at any medical school. The Community Service Initiative is a good, specific program for this medical school, but the student needs to effectively highlight their own experiences as to why this is important for them. They do, on the other hand, try to "sell"*

> *what they consider to be skills important for a good physician—*
> *sensitivity and genuine kindness to those in need. Don't make your*
> *responses a sales pitch for the skills you think are important. Stick to*
> *answering the prompt.*

What is the nature of your interest in the ABC School of Medicine?

There are many reasons why I am so attracted to the idea of learning medicine at ABC School of Medicine. Coming from multiple rural communities, I value the ability to develop strong, long-lasting relationships. The longitudinal faculty-student relationships promoted at the ABC School of Medicine are a driving factor for my interest. I feel the ability to connect at that level with those teaching me would provide an enhanced overall learning experience. This summer I performed research on a multidisciplinary headache clinic, involving neurology, behavioral health, and nutrition. I worked closely with all providers involved and learned about the benefits and challenges they face working this closely across departments, and found it to be both interesting and convenient for the patient. The focus on interdisciplinary training at ABC School of Medicine would provide me with the excellent learning opportunity to continue exploring this type of collaboration that will likely be prevalent in my future. Growing up, working, and shadowing in medically underserved communities, I was exposed to the negative impact that inaccessibility to adequate healthcare had on those around me. I am extremely interested in getting involved in the Bridging the Gaps program to aid those underserved people. I feel the opportunity to participate in this program would help me learn more about this topic and continue my passion to assist this population in my practice of medicine someday. I'm also interested in the ability to train with the Emergency Action Corps in disaster response. My family is what one may label as "preppers," a group of people who prepare for a variety of potential life-altering disasters. The ability to combine my interests in medicine and responses to a large-scale tragedy is an opportunity I strive to pursue. Each of these I would be extremely grateful to utilize as a medical student at the ABC School of Medicine.

This is a very good response to a "Why this medical school?" prompt. At each point, the student was able to reflect on their specific journey. Discussing their family as "preppers" gives the reader a visual and supports why the student is interested in disaster response. Talking about growing up in a medically underserved area, the student supports their interest in the Bridging the Gaps program. Each point was supported and not just copied and pasted from the school's website.

How did you learn about osteopathic medicine?

While working as a nurse in a rehab facility, I met Dr. Brown who is an osteopathic physician. I was covering some of their patients that day, in particular "Mr. Larry." Mr. Larry was new to the rehab facility and was complaining of sleep problems being in unfamiliar territory and requested something to help him sleep. Dr. Brown assessed him and ordered melatonin to aid, but Mr. Larry did not want to take melatonin because he thought that an over the counter medication will not work as well as a prescribed medication. I watched Dr. Brown take the time to educate Mr. Larry on the melatonin uses and he finally agreed to try it. When I followed up with him a few weeks later, he was ecstatic because he got sufficient rest as result of the melatonin. I began to realize that osteopathic medicine was unique and utilized a different mindset and that was the initial peak of interest into osteopathic medicine. Furthermore, the uniqueness, integration and introduction of various influences that can affect the patient and treatment plan in the practice of clinical medicine has been a key reason of my pursuit of osteopathic medicine.

While it's great that the student is trying to tell the story of a patient interaction with an osteopathic physician, the example doesn't really point out any of the traditional osteopathic philosophies. I would try to highlight those philosophies and what they mean to you when discussing your exposure to osteopathic medicine. However, do not just list the philosophies—separate them and reflect on them.

SITUATIONAL JUDGMENT TESTS

S ituational judgment tests, or SJTs, are tests that present the test taker with realistic, hypothetical situations. For the purposes of the medical school application, you need to be aware of two SJTs: CASPer and the aptly named AAMC SJT.

CASPer

What is CASPer?

CASPer (Computer-Based Assessment for Sampling Personal Characteristics) was co-created and developed by Altus Assessments, which is the same team (from McMaster University) that blessed us with the multiple mini-interview (MMI). For a great discussion about CASPer with co-creator Dr. Kelly Dore, check out Session 303 of *The Premed Years* podcast at premedyears.com/303 and an updated conversation during National Premed Day 2020 at mappd.tv.

CASPer is a form of a situational judgment test used to present you with different types of scenarios to assess what you would do in each of the situations.

Situational judgment tests try to figure out what you will do and how you will behave in each of the situations presented. Many students say the experience is similar to a five-minute MMI. According to Altus Assessments, they are assessing for collaboration, communication, empathy, equity, ethics, motivation, problem solving, professionalism, resilience, and self-awareness. These qualities are hard to assess in a traditional interview format or anywhere else in an application.

What is on CASPer?

CASPer is made up of 12 different sections, with each section containing a video or written scenario and three open-ended questions. You'll have a total of five-minutes for your responses to the three questions. CASPer takes 60 to 90 minutes to complete, with an optional 15-minute break half-way through. Unlike an MCAT, in which there are right and wrong answers, CASPer is scored by humans who work for Altus Assessments. A different rater scores each section of the test based on set criteria for each scenario.

Which Schools Use CASPer?

You should go to takecasper.com to see which schools use CASPer. New schools are added every year, so make sure to check the site around the time of your application.

Preparing for CASPer

CASPer doesn't require any specific preparation outside of understanding the test. If you do a web search for "how to prepare for CASPer," you will find programs and companies out there selling services to help you prepare for CASPer. Be that as it may, you don't need to do this since Altus Assessments provides free test prep on their site at takecasper.com.

Ultimately, the best preparation for CASPer is just to be a good human being and be yourself. One student said it best when I was talking about CASPer during a Facebook Live session: "Don't be a psychopath, and you'll be fine."

There is no shortage of example scenarios online if you want to look for more. You will find that common questions in the situation presented to you are

"How would you handle this situation?", "Do you think this is right?", "What advice would you give?", or "Tell us of a time…."

How is CASPer Scored?

A different rater, who is unaware of your personal information, reviews each scenario. What the raters are specifically looking for is obviously unknown. In the end, you are given a raw score that is converted to a z-score, where 0 is the mean. Scores are normalized for the specific test you took on that particular date and time. Any red flags in your answer are marked and reviewed. The score will not mean anything to you, but it will help the medical schools see how you compare to other applicants who applied to their school.

Do I Have to Type Fast?

One of the biggest complaints of CASPer is that it is a timed test, and you have to type a lot. Students who type slowly may complain because they don't have enough time to input all of the information they think is needed. You need to be able to type well and type fast, but you don't have to be the world's fastest typist. You also don't need to worry about making sure everything is grammatically correct and/or spelled correctly, as you're not scored on that.

There is also not a specific format that is required or even frowned upon. Find the format that works best for you to explain yourself. If that means you are typing in paragraphs, great. If you need to use bullet points, that is okay, too. As long as your thoughts get out there.

When Do I Take CASPer?

You need to take CASPer early on in the application cycle. Depending on the school, if CASPer is part of the secondary application process, they may not consider your application complete until your CASPer score is received by the medical school, which can take about three weeks.

Because of rolling admissions, you want to make sure your CASPer score is submitted as soon as possible so your application can be completed earlier and you can be reviewed for a potential interview.

Looking at the previous application cycle, it appears CASPer tests students applying to medical school between the months of May and December.

Where Do I Take CASPer?

CASPer is taken at home on your own computer. You will need to have a functional webcam that must be active, uncovered, and facing you when you are taking the test. Altus Assessments has a list of system requirements that you should review early enough to make any necessary accommodations. While you do need to be dressed, you do not need to be formally dressed up for the test.

Will I Get my Score?

As this book is being written, Altus is working on sending students their scores. Prior to this, scores were not sent out to students. Right now, only a subset of students is receiving their scores. In the future, all students may receive their scores.

How Much Does CASPer Cost?

The current fee to take CASPer is $10, with an additional $10 to submit to each medical school that requires CASPer. CASPer does waive your fees if you are approved for the Fee Assistance Program from the AAMC or AACOM. You should check takecasper.com for the most up-to-date fees.

Rescheduling CASPer

You can reschedule CASPer at any point prior to your test for free, as long as there are dates and times available. You can also reschedule if you missed your scheduled test date and time as long as you have not seen any content.

How is CASPer Used?

Every medical school that requests CASPer as part of their application process may use it in a different way. Some medical schools use it as a sole secondary application with no other essay questions needed, while others use it in addition to secondary essays.

Some schools may use CASPer to determine who is invited for an interview. Some schools may be using CASPer after an interview as part of their review process to see who they want to accept. CASPer might also be used for data purposes to see how CASPer lines up with accepted students to determine if the school wants to use CASPer more prominently in the future.

At the end of the day, you cannot control how the medical schools are going to use the CASPer score, so you really should not waste a lot of time thinking about it. Understand it, take it, and move on to the rest of your application.

AAMC SJT

What is the AAMC SJT?

The AAMC SJT is a new test created by the AAMC and tested at a couple of medical schools during the 2020-2021 application cycle. As of the writing of this book, it is still too early to know if it will be offered moving forward.

Similar to CASPer, the AAMC SJT is based on realistic, hypothetical situations that a student may encounter during or after medical school to assess a student's pre-professional competencies.

The biggest difference between the AAMC SJT and CASPer is how responses are submitted. CASPer responses are typed by students, while AAMC SJT is a multiple-choice test.

What is on the AAMC SJT?

The AAMC SJT contains 30 scenarios with 186 questions. Similar to the MCAT, the AAMC SJT contains experimental questions that won't be scored. Each response asks you to rate it from 1 (very ineffective) to 4 (very effective). The AAMC SJT takes 75 minutes to complete, with a total time of about 100 minutes to complete the entire SJT session.

Which Schools Use the AAMC SJT?

At the time of this writing, the AAMC SJT was being tested at the University of California Davis School of Medicine and the University of Minnesota Medical

School Twin Cities campus. Check the AAMC website for the most current list of schools using the AAMC SJT.

Preparing for the AAMC SJT

Similar to the CASPer, you don't need any specific preparation to do well on the AAMC SJT. The AAMC provides a practice exam, which you can find on the AAMC site at students-residents.aamc.org.

How is the AAMC SJT Scored?

Students are given a score from 1 to 9, as well as a percentile rank that shows the percentages of students who scored at the same score or lower. If you void your exam on your test day, you will not receive a score, nor will the medical schools.

When to Take the AAMC SJT

During this first testing year, the AAMC SJT was offered during two windows. Both windows were over six days at the beginning of September. Please check the AAMC website for exam dates for your cycle.

Where Do I Take the AAMC SJT?

The AAMC SJT is taken at home on your own computer. Your computer must have a functional webcam. The AAMC has a list of technical requirements that you should review early enough to make any necessary accommodations.

Will I Get my Score?

The AAMC will release your AAMC SJT score to you. You will receive an email when it's released with instructions on how to view it.

How Much Does the AAMC SJT Cost?

At the time of this writing, the AAMC SJT is free. I would expect that to change in the future.

Rescheduling the AAMC SJT

You can reschedule the AAMC SJT until the registration deadline of your current exam date. Pay attention to these details when you register.

How is the AAMC SJT Used?

At the time of this writing, the two schools piloting the AAMC SJT are reviewing how the AAMC SJT scores will help in each's holistic review process. It is too soon to know exactly how schools will use them, but like everything else, each medical school will determine how they want to use the scores in their admissions process.

INTERVIEWS

I f you've gotten to this point in the application process and you have received an interview to medical school, then you are doing something right. You have shown at least one medical school your reasons for wanting to be a physician, and they like your reasons and your story. You have shown them your academic capabilities with your GPA and your MCAT, and the scores are acceptable to them. You have filled out your secondary applications and turned them around in a timely manner, and/or you have taken the CASPer/AAMC SJT and scored well. Plus, you gathered either a committee letter or letters of recommendations from professors, physicians, and anyone else who has shown the Admissions Committee your character and who you are as a person. You've done everything right to this point to be able to get an interview. If you look at the averages, only about 5% of applicants get an interview at each particular school. Now your goal is to prepare for the interview so you can turn that interview invite into an acceptance.

The interview day is your opportunity to show the Admissions Committee you are a normal human being who can hold a conversation. You also need to show how you will be a good classmate, teammate, and colleague in the future.

Just as the personal statement is not your opportunity to sell your skills on why you think you're going to be a great physician, neither is the interview.

You may be questioning: "But Dr. Gray, how are they going to know I'm going to be a great physician if I can't tell them I'm going to be a great physician?" Just stop and think about that question for one second. Do you think you are the only student who has ever thought, "Man, I really need to tell these people that I'm going to be a great physician. Nobody else is going to think about saying that, and that is going to separate me and make me a more valuable candidate." Does that sound logical? It doesn't to me, and it shouldn't to you, either.

Your job on interview day is to show up on time, dress well, be friendly and professional to everyone, and have real and honest conversations. Show them who you are as a person by communicating with them. When they ask you to tell them about yourself, a very common opening question in a traditional interview format, your job isn't to say, "Well, I went to the University of Florida, and I majored in biochemistry and I got a 3.9 GPA, and I was the president of the premed club, and I have 3000 hours of research experience, and I'm really dedicated to the community. I was part of Big Brothers and Big Sisters, and I've known I wanted to be a doctor forever. Oh, I also have tons of shadowing experience, and I'm just… I know that with my skills as a good communicator and as an empathetic person that I'm going to make a great physician, and I just want the opportunity."

That's how a lot of students answer that question. But what if we did it a different way, and you actually just showed who you are as a person? Instead, you can state, "Well, I grew up in California, and when I was 12, I moved to Florida after the Rodney King riots. I played baseball as a kid, and I was pretty talented, and I thought I was going to play in college and hopefully beyond. But I injured my shoulder playing baseball in high school. I still love baseball, and I still play to this day in men's adult leagues. I have a brother, and I really love computers, computer programming, and podcasting. I love listening to podcasts, especially business podcasts, but my favorite is Radiolab. I also love traveling. I've been to Kenya and would love to go back someday to see the big game animals. I'd also love to travel to other parts of the world as I grow up and have more means to do that. One of my favorite things to do right now is to cook. I've been trying to perfect a spaghetti recipe with my brother for years, and I think we're getting close to doing that. That's a little bit about me."

Now the interviewer has a picture in their mind of who you are as a person, not just an interviewee. You're someone who likes sports, who loves to cook and make spaghetti, and who likes to travel. Maybe your interviewer has been to Kenya before, and after mentioning your trip there, they can say, "Oh, Kenya, where did you go? Which parks did you visit? Which animals did you see? What's your favorite animal? Oh, you like cooking spaghetti. I love spaghetti; I have to eat gluten-free noodles, though, because I have celiac disease."

With the second example, you're connecting to another human being through a conversation. That is the goal of the interview. Just like with the personal statements, I've written a whole book on the interview process, and I highly encourage you to get a copy of that book anywhere books are sold by searching for *The Premed Playbook: Guide to the Medical School Interview*. In that book, there are over 600 questions that can give you an idea of what to be prepared for on interview day. You can also go onto my website at medicalschoolhq.net and click on "Tools," and then click on the Medical School Interview Question Generator.

The Anti-Goal of the Interview

While writing this book, I had a lot of conversations with students who have been on an interview and felt like it didn't go well. I want to highlight one of those conversations for you here—about what *not* to do.

I spoke with a student who wasn't getting any acceptances after his medical school interview. I wanted to dig in and find out why.

While talking about the interviews he attended, he specifically mentioned one that he felt went well. The student talked about being truly himself because he was able to answer every question honestly and through the lens of his passion for medicine. **This was a major red flag for me.**

I dug in even deeper, trying to understand what he meant by this. After some back and forth, I was finally able to understand what he meant. He used the example of "What do you do in your free time?" With this answer, he told the interviewer what he did in his free time **while also** relating it back to medicine in some way.

DO NOT DO THIS.

When an interviewer asks you about what you do in your free time, they want to know what you do in your free time. They do not want to know about how everything in your life ties back to medicine. This is a very common mistake that students make.

Your goal is to have a conversation with the interviewer, not twist everything around like a politician to fit a narrative you think is important.

Preparing for the Interview

Even though there are many questions in my interview book to prepare for, the goal of preparing for the interview isn't to be able to answer all of those questions or every question you think will come up; rather, it is to be comfortable reacting and talking about anything asked. In fact, the more you practice your answers, the worse you will likely do because you will be over-rehearsed.

The more you practice just being comfortable answering anything, the better your interview day will go, as you'll sound more natural. As soon as you can, talk with your pre-health advisor or whomever does mock interviews on your campus, and start the process of mock interviewing with them.

Luckily, interviewing is a skill you can learn, assuming you get proper feedback and you implement that feedback to improve. Be prepared to get feedback you might not agree with or that you feel is critical. Understand the criticism is there to help you improve your communication style so that on interview day, you can show the Admissions Committee who you are, instead of stressing about the interview process and performing poorly.

Types of Interviews

There are many different types of interviews you may find on the interview trail. The preparation for each may vary, but ultimately the foundation is the same—be yourself.

Traditional Interview

The traditional interview is a one-on-one interview with someone who has been selected and trained to interview prospective students. The interviewer could be a faculty member, a medical student, or somebody from the community who has volunteered to interview students.

The traditional interview can be open-file, closed-file, or partially open (sometimes referred to as partially closed).

The following are common traditional interview questions:

- Tell me about yourself.
- Why do you want to be a doctor?
- What is your greatest strength?
- What is your biggest weakness?
- Why should we accept you?
- Do you think the US should have a single-payer healthcare system?
- Why do you want to come to this school?
- Tell me about a time you failed and what you learned from it.

Open-file Interview

An open-file interview means the interviewer has access to all of your information, including your essays and grades.

As with every interview, for an open-file interview, you should be intimately familiar with every aspect of your application, both primary and secondary. You need to be prepared to handle any questions that come directly from your application, including any red flags such as institutional actions, poor grades, or gaps in your activities.

Just because the interviewer has access to those things doesn't mean they've actually looked at them. Avoid using statements like, "As you've seen in my personal statement," since you don't know what they have or have not read to this point.

One of the biggest mistakes I see students making with open-file interviews is avoiding the "best answer" during questioning because they already told that story or gave that answer in their application, and they don't want to repeat themselves. Don't be afraid of repeating what is in your application unless you are specifically told otherwise. Changing who you are or giving a weaker answer to avoid repetition will only make your interview weaker than it should be.

Closed-file Interview

A closed-file interview, also referred to as a blind interview, is an interview in which the interviewer doesn't have access to any of the information in your application. I believe you should approach a closed-file interview and an open-file interview in the same exact way. The biggest difference is the interviewer won't be picking questions directly out of your application in a closed-file interview.

The biggest mistake I see students making with closed-file interviews is trying to include parts of their application, even if it's not part of the question, because they feel they only have one opportunity to show the interviewer how compassionate they are because the interviewer has not seen their application. Answer the question that is being asked without adding in your own "agenda."

Politicians are very good at answering questions in this way: "Thank you for the question, and here is what I really want to talk about..." If you are taking each question and trying to figure out how to spin it with your strengths, don't. This is good advice for every interview style, but particularly for closed-file interviews.

Partially-Closed/Partially-Blind Interview

A partially-closed or partially-blind interview is one in which the interviewer typically has access to your essays and possibly your extracurriculars, but not your grades. This is to remove any sort of bias, such as if you potentially have a low MCAT score or a low GPA. This could help remove a negative opinion of you.

Multiple Mini Interview (MMI)

The Multiple Mini Interview, also known as the MMI, is a new interview format started at McMaster University in Canada by the same people who later created the CASPer test. The MMI is similar to the CASPer in that they are both situational tests in which you answer questions or engage in scenarios with an interviewer, actor, or another student. Common MMI scenarios include moral and ethical debates, dealing with tough patients, giving news to patients, or working through building a LEGO car with another student.

The MMI is implemented differently at every school, so every MMI that you go through may be a little bit different. Some schools use part MMI and part traditional interview. Some schools may use just the MMI, while others may have traditional interview questions mixed into MMI stations without a separate traditional interview.

You have to be prepared for anything on your interview day. Once you learn what the MMI is about and what it is for, it should be a fun experience for you. The goal of the MMI, just like the traditional interview, is to test your communication skills and your thought process. Again, the goal is not to give the "perfect" answers or to show you are an amazing human being; it is to assess your verbal and nonverbal skills through interaction.

MMI Format

A traditional MMI format includes seven to ten "stations," with a different scenario at each station. At each station, you are typically given two minutes to stand outside the room and read the scenario before an audible alarm goes off to let you know you can enter the room. Inside the room, there will either be an interviewer, an actor and a reviewer, or some other group of people to work with based on the scenario. You will typically have six to eight minutes inside of the room to work through that scenario. You don't have to talk the whole time. The goal of the MMI is to answer the questions posed in the scenario and then to allow the interviewer to ask you follow-up questions. Again, every school is different, and some schools don't have their interviewers ask follow-up questions. Try to get a feel for the school you are interviewing at and see what they expect.

The goal with the actor-based scenarios is to make sure you leave plenty of time to listen because this is the most important part of communication. If you are given a scenario in which there is an upset patient (the actor), listen to them first, then find out why the patient is upset and ask questions to elicit those responses. Always listen to those responses; do not just think about the next question you want to ask. The MMI is complete once you have rotated through all of the stations.

Here is an example MMI scenario:

You are a trainer at your local gym. Today, you are covering at the front desk, greeting visitors, and responding to questions from patrons. One of the patrons approaches the counter. They are clearly angry about something, though you're not quite sure what happened to upset them, as their rant is unclear. Before you are able to respond, they become increasingly aggressive toward you personally. How do you respond?

Benefits of the MMI

Unlike a traditional interview in which you might have two one-on-one interviews, the MMI affords you the ability to make a mistake in one station but still save your interview day by doing well in the other stations. If you err in a traditional one-on-one interview, and you only have two interviewers that day, there's a good chance you will not get into that medical school. The MMI is meant to test multiple non-cognitive abilities, and its goal is to remove a lot of interview bias and subjectivity from the process.

Interview Timeline

As I wrote about in the application timeline, interviews can start around mid- to late-July and continue into late March or even April. The DO timeline has historically been a bit more drawn out than the MD application, so you may see students getting interviews later if they are interviewing at DO schools. The same is true for very early interviews since DO applications are transmitted to schools before MD applications.

Once offered an interview, medical schools usually give you the opportunity to pick different available dates. Remember, because of rolling admissions, the earlier you interview, the earlier (typically) you will be evaluated for an acceptance. Choosing an earlier interview date may potentially help you when it comes to getting an acceptance.

Virtual Interviews

Pre-COVID-19, the majority of medical schools would not allow virtual interviews. It will be interesting to see what happens moving forward. To the best of your ability, do not plan to take a vacation or any trips during the application season. If you're a nontraditional student and you have a job and/ or responsibilities, you may not be able to dictate that in your schedule. Try to communicate those issues and what you will need during this time with your employer. This gets a little more difficult if you are hiding the fact that you are applying to medical school from your supervisor or employer. I hid this fact from my supervisor, only to find out her father was a Pulmonologist on the Admissions Committee at WashU. Oops! I recommend finding someone you can confide in who will help you navigate what you need at work as you are going through the application cycle.

What to Bring

On your interview day, the only thing you really have to bring is yourself. I recommend bringing some sort of folio with paper and a pen to take notes. You don't need to bring your transcripts, résumés, or applications since the medical school will have all of that information.

You may get a random interviewer who was added at the last minute and may not have access to your application, but that's okay, as they will access it afterward. Definitely *do not* bring your phone to the interview day. If you have to have it on you, turn it off completely. The last thing you want to have happen is for your phone to go off while the Dean of Admissions is presenting information about the school to a roomful of interviewees. That is a very easy way to ensure you will not get an acceptance to that medical school.

What to Wear

The medical school interview is a professional interview; thus, everyone should dress in business attire. Men should wear a suit, including a tie (you can rock a bow tie if you want). Women might wear a dress with a cardigan, but I don't think that is formal enough. A pant suit, dress suit, or skirt suit is suitable for an interview.

You want to be remembered on your interview day, but not for the wrong reasons, such as attire. Standing out on the interview day because you wore a light blue suit is probably not a good idea, nor is wearing your power red suit. Black, brown, navy, and charcoal-colored suits are better choices. You should not use a lot of makeup or have a shocking hair color either.

Remove any sort of body accessories that may distract others or make them question your professionalism. You have to remember that a large majority of your interviewers are probably from another generation and aren't accustomed to seeing, or maybe aren't comfortable with, tattoos and piercings. As someone with three tattoos, I'm all for them, but make sure to cover them up as best you can on your interview day.

If you do enjoy body modifications and crazy hair colors, make sure you get a hold of the student handbook to see what is allowed if you are accepted to the school.

Pre-interview Parties

Some medical schools have a dinner or reception the night before the interview. I always get questions from students if they should plan to go to these, and the answer is always, "100%, yes!"

The goal of this whole process, and the goal in life in general, is to build your network and your connections. A pre-interview reception, where you will meet medical students, fellow interviewees, and others, is your opportunity to connect and relax before your interview day. Meeting those people, seeing their faces, and recognizing them on the interview day will lower your stress level because you've already interacted with them. You will also realize they are not there to attack you, but really just to get to know you. Make arrangements to go to those parties, as it might pay off in the end.

Follow the dress code for these types of events as well. If the dress code is casual, dress well, but don't go in a suit. If there is no dress code given, default to business casual.

Remember that every interaction may make its way back to the Admissions Committee, so you always want to be on your best behavior.

Travel Arrangements

Most interview days take up a large portion of the day, and you will most likely not leave town until either really late that night or the next day. Also, plan on arriving the day *before* your interview. Do not try to manage to get there super early in the morning if the interview starts a little bit later in the day. Get there and be comfortable, so you don't have to worry about your plane being late and missing your interview. If you can, and you have the time, take a practice trip to the school and find out where the interview will be so that on the interview day, you are not concerned about getting lost on campus.

Post-interview Thank You Letters

I highly recommend sending thank you letters either directly to the interviewer or to the Admissions Committee in general. I would find out from the medical school if they prefer emails or physical letters.

Try to send your thank you notes as soon as possible, the same day, preferably. Additionally, take notes after every encounter about something potentially memorable that happened that you can bring up in your thank you note. If you got into a conversation with your interviewer about the New York Yankees and how you both have a love for them, maybe you can mention that you are rooting for the Yankees, and you hope they pull through this year.

There are some schools that will tell you not to send any thank you letters, and you should follow their recommendations. As with everything, every school and every Admissions Committee differs. My recommendation is to default to sending a letter, even if it is not going to impact anything.

Examples

Below are examples from real mock interviews I held with students specifically for this book. I focused on common questions you might get during your interviews. For more examples, check out my other book, *The Premed Playbook: Guide to the Medical School Interview,* and look for more mock interviews coming to my YouTube channel at premed.tv.

Most questions below are answered by multiple students designated "Student A," "Student B," etc. You should not assume "Student A" is the same student for two different questions. Also, an ellipsis (…) in these answers is not where I've removed part of the answer. These are breaks in the student's thoughts.

What Do You Think is the Biggest Challenge that Physicians Will Face in Ten Years?

Student A

Student A: I think from where we used to be a couple years ago, and to my understanding of 27 years of life on this planet and maybe nine- to 10- year journey of being a premed student, I feel like things are getting better as far as medicine goes, as far as the healthcare system. It might not be the most perfect, but I feel like it is getting somewhat better than where we used to be. I feel physician burnout is improving, as far as advocacy for it. Being more aware of it, so I feel in that aspect of it, things are progressing better in that sense. Then also like in academia and academic medicine I feel like there's a lot more transparency and ability to be able to talk, and speak out, about certain things. With cutting back and limiting residency hours for residents, things are improving.

So, I'm projecting that the field will be getting better, whether it be for physicians, or for patients, and for the healthcare system that we have. I predict the future, potentially, we build a system that might be able to address whatever shortcomings we have now in the current healthcare system. We might have more support, more resources for physicians as we progress, to reduce burnout. Whether it be more combined sub-specialties, residency programs where physicians can do combine anesthesia or EM, which gives them an ability to have a different lifestyle and different life in hospital, and clinic. So, they wouldn't have to be just one specialty, which tends to be burning out.

I think as far as academia goes and the medical school system is there's a lot more support, and a lot more mental health, and a lot more resources for students to succeed in and out of the classroom. So, I think in the long run it will be getting better for everybody involved.

Dr. Gray: All right, but the question was what will be the biggest challenge for a physician in 10 years. You didn't answer that question.

Student A: Sorry. Sorry. I thought you said, "What do you see it being in the future better?" Sorry.

The biggest challenge, I think, for physicians would be I think just learning the nuances and the intricacies of the healthcare system, and how it works, and how it's always changing. How a lot of us, whether it be pre-med, or medical students, or physicians, don't really have a good understanding of the healthcare system because all we do is study the science. I think the biggest challenge would be able to continue fighting those battles with the healthcare aspect of it and the politics aspect of it. But I'm hopeful that with more awareness we become more of advocates for both ourselves and our patients.

Dr. Gray: Awesome. How is that different than right now?

Student A: Well, I mean I think it is one of the biggest challenges to date and there always has been that battle between the healthcare administration on a system base, and the physician and trying to just treat the patient. I think it's always been like that and it continues to be like that. I feel like it's getting better, like I formerly mentioned, but I feel like that's always going to be a challenge that can still exist. But it will be reduced, hopefully one day, to just completely be eliminated and everybody being 100% understanding of it.

> *This student started off by answering the wrong question. Make sure you are listening during your interview. It is unacceptable to answer the wrong question. After being redirected, the student gave a decent answer, but I challenged them a little because I was not sure their response was any different than the current situation. If the student had mentioned it was a similar struggle right now, it would have shown some awareness of the current struggles and their expectation that it was going to continue to be a struggle.*

Student B

Student B: In 10 years, I would say, depending on the changes with the payer systems, and insurances, and Medicare, if that changes, that will be definitely a big issue for them. Otherwise, I think still fighting the opioid epidemic, and I think just a lot of the ethical stuff that's still going on now is still going to be a problem then, because you can't satisfy everyone on all fronts.

And I think medicine is still very political, even though you try to separate it. We still butt heads a lot with the business aspect of medicine, and I think that that's going to be one of the bigger challenges for us, is just trying to find common ground, and making sure that our medical model expresses what we think medicine should be as physicians, and how we ensure social justice while still keeping a sustainable practice and sustainable hospital systems.

> *The question is, "What is the biggest challenge?" and the student listed a bunch of different things. Some aspects of the answer were more focused on negative things, like butting heads with the business aspect of medicine. While true, this could have been worded a little differently to avoid the negativity in the answer itself. In relation to answering the question, the student listed several different things, which made them struggle to focus on answering the question. Make sure you answer the question.*

Student C

Student C: You know, the biggest challenge for physicians in 10 years is probably finding the right people to... Excuse me, let me think about that for a second.

Dr. Gray: Okay.

Student C: You know, with all of the technology that everyone has access to now, I guess the biggest challenge in 10 years might be that kind of trust between physicians and patients. Patients may think that Dr. Google has all the answers, whereas the physicians who train actually do have that information. And you know, that kind of physician-patient trust may be compromised, because the patients might receive different information from different sources, and not initially trust the physician exactly.

> *This is an interesting answer. The Dr. Google debate typically comes from a point of frustration with physicians, to say, "Why don't patients believe me? Why are patients doing all of this research and coming to me with a diagnosis already?" And it's coming, typically, from a place of frustration and being jaded towards patients. So, it's interesting that the answer is focused on this because most premed students are too young to have this potentially jaded point of view*

already. I'd be careful with that answer. I think we will potentially always have a situation where patients are going to want to do their own research to try to understand what's going on with their bodies, and as physicians, we need to be open and accepting of that.

This answer potentially gives off a vibe that the student wants to always be trusted and doesn't want to be questioned. Your answers have a lot of power, so make sure you understand what you're saying.

In addition, the student started their answer and then stopped. Always take a second to think about how you're going to respond, rather than rushing ahead. When you drive to a new destination, you don't want to get half-way there and realize you're going in the wrong direction. It's never wrong to ask for a second to compose your answers in your mind before answering, but don't do it for every question. A quick pause is usually enough for students to gather their thoughts.

How Would You Fix Rising Drug Costs?

Student A

Student A: That's a tough thing to look at because the healthcare system is really, really complex. There's a lot of modalities that go into it, but if I had to choose a way to fix it and reduce costs, I think it would be maybe using some of the… I'm trying to think of the word. But I know that, from my understanding of the healthcare system, there are certain credits that the government will give to certain pharmaceutical companies or insurance companies to reduce costs and whatnot. So, my understanding, if some of those things would be used to… That would normally be used maybe for say to reduce… Pretty much could be used to reduce the cost of pharmaceuticals. I think it could definitely reduce the cost.

Also, I know that working in clinical trials myself as a coordinator I know that… Now understanding the amount of research and the amount of work that goes into devices or drug trials, I understand why the cost is so expensive for these medications or for these devices. I think maybe finding ways to work with the FDA to not reduce regulations but find better alternatives to make those things be more expedited, that still doesn't put the patient's safety at risk, could really reduce those costs. The amount of investigation work that goes into it.

The last thing I would probably think about would be maybe seeing if there are different alternatives to… As far as drug development, using different things that are using the chemicals to make it. Like different alternatives to make substitutions to be cheaper. Like more cost-effective. My predicament is how we go about it, but I'm not 100% sure.

> *The student did a good job with their thought process, which is the goal of these questions. You're not supposed to have the* right *answer; you're just supposed to talk through your thoughts. This student did that. One thing I mentioned to the student was that their idea of "credits" isn't really reducing the cost but just shifting around who is paying for it. This is a very common answer when talking about reducing costs—students focus on shifting the burden. Hopefully, this provides some information to formulate a better answer in your interviews.*

Student B

Student B: I think that it's incredibly important to ensure that there are cost controls within the government, but I'm not sure I see that happening without some basic changes, such as being able to limit contributions to campaigns within the political system, such as controlling how we do lobbying, that without some of these basic political changes, we're going to continue to have this price gouging. I mean, look at what happened with Martin Shkreli, that when people with insane amounts of wealth are able to have all the power they do, that they can really do whatever they want with drug prices. And so, I believe the only way to really combat that is to fight the corruption in the system so we can actually lay out a system that works. But before we get to that point, it's impossible to implement anything.

Dr. Gray: There are some states that are looking at becoming pharmaceutical companies themselves to start making generic medications for people who live in their states, and there are people who want to buy medications from other countries like Canada, where the cost for the same medication is significantly cheaper. Do you think those are valid alternatives?

Student B: I would say that I have some concerns off the bat, being that we already have a good amount of difference in how state-run programs are able to implement things such as education. And while I'm very attracted to the idea of being able to moderate some of those prices, I'd really need to see that, before a state went ahead with something like that, that the alternatives were really sound, that they weren't in some way creating larger issues.

The student had a great thought process behind these answers. I gave a follow-up question because the student seemed to understand the political system a little more than many other students. This is a perfect example of how being yourself and giving your answer can flow into a conversation with the interviewer. I wasn't planning on asking the follow-up question, but it worked really well after their initial answer.

Why Osteopathic Medicine?

Student A

Student A: As a powerlifter, I've been working with different physical therapists and chiropractors and massage therapists. So, I'm actually very interested in how physical medicine and the osteopathic manipulative medicine could offer individuals benefits for chronic pain or for sports injuries or issues that they may be having to work through. I think it kind of brings a different tool that I could use to help patients, which I don't see that in any way being a negative thing. I would probably still be interested in it even if I went to an MD school. I know you can go to osteopathic manipulative medicine, like training even as an MD.

Dr. Gray: Have you had any experience with a DO at all?

Student A: I have not seen one for physical issues where I needed manipulative medicine work. I used to see one as my family care practitioner. I also scribed for a DO in the emergency department, but they were not able to do OMT in the emergency department. I've asked them about how they would use it. They've brought up cases for chronic pain patients that we see all the time that are like, oh, if I had a table, I could fix them right here and now. But I don't know if that would make the answer stronger or not.

I really like how this student brought in their own experience as a powerlifter and what they've experienced working with physical therapy and massage therapy. While not directly associated with osteopathic medicine, it shows an understanding of how different modalities can treat a patient.

After I asked whether or not the student had any experience with a DO, they had a gold mine of information that could have added to their original answer. Having been cared for by a DO and shadowing a DO shows more insight into the osteopathic world.

You can see how the student was able to answer the question without bringing up the cliché "holistic philosophy" that many students lean on as a crutch for this question. All physicians treat their patients holistically, not just osteopathic physicians.

Student B

Student B: I definitely agree or believe in the holistic approach to medicine. I want to view the patient in that holistic view and treating them the best way possible. I know that MD or allopathic medicine takes that approach as well, but it's more common with the DO practice.

You can see that this example is the opposite of the previous one. No personal connection. No thought process. This is just the cliché "holistic philosophy" that students use. If you want to bring up holistic philosophy, try to expand on what holistic means and why it's important to you. And if you're interviewing at an osteopathic medical school, don't say, "Well, I know MDs do it, too." Again, if you have any experience seeing osteopathic physicians yourself, shadowing them, or seeing OMT, make sure you mention that and its impact on you.

Student C

Student C: I saw my first DO when I was, I guess, early adulthood, and I'd never seen one before, but it was for muscle joint pain. And she asked me if she could perform osteopathic manipulative medicine on me, and I didn't really know what that was. I was familiar with chiropractors at that point, but not DOs or OMM. I'd actually seen a DO prior to that, I think, but OMM wasn't offered. So, she did the OMM treatment on me, and it was amazing, and her bedside manner I felt was very different from what I'd experienced in the past. She listens more, and took into account my whole story, instead of just focusing on illness or disability-type stuff. She kind of went a little further and dug a little deeper into it, and at that point I was already a nurse, and I just, I felt like the whole appointment went differently, and it was a pretty amazing experience to me. So, I've tried to learn a little bit more about that and how it differs from an MD practice.

> *I like how this student was able to bring in a personal experience. Your personal experiences will almost always make your answers stronger. This borders a little bit on saying that DOs are better than MDs. It is very common for students to say that osteopathic physicians care more, listen more, dig deeper, etc.; however, it is important to remember that every physician differs, and being a good listener and digging deeper isn't unique to osteopathic physicians. Outside of your personal experience, try to be objective with your answer.*

Student D

Student D: You know, osteopathic medicine, I've heard that osteopaths learn a little bit different things than allopaths do in medical school. And you know, I think that's a very valuable trait to have. If I'm going down this road, I want to be exposed to all aspects of medicine, not just a single viewpoint. So, I think that the OMT that osteopaths learn is very valuable and can be applied in many ways that allopaths can't.

Dr. Gray: Have you had any exposure to osteopathic medicine, to OMT at all?

Student D: I have not. I've been looking out and reaching out to a few osteopaths through cold calls, but I have had no success with that so far.

> *This answer was a little brief and didn't show any sort of understanding other than "it's different." To me, this student likely hasn't done any research into osteopathic medicine. The answer is very superficial. Try to expand as much as possible to show your comprehension and what you've researched. Even if you haven't been able to shadow or see OMT, you can address that. You can say you've tried (if you truly have), which shows interest. As a side note, I personally do not like to refer to osteopathic physicians as "osteopaths." Osteopathy is a different field in the majority of the rest of the world.*

Tell Me About a Time You Failed

Student A

Student A: Oh, my entire undergraduate career. And in terms of my broadest goal, I went into undergraduate career wanting to get into medical school but not necessarily appreciating how competitive it was to get in.

I was a smart kid all through elementary, middle school, high school. People kept telling me that getting into college is going to be hard. It was going to be a challenge, and I kind of read through it and got into the college I wanted. And I hit undergrad, and I failed a class my freshman year, and that was terrible, and I was like, "You know, okay. I was just being a bit of a dumb freshman. These things happen." And I ended up turning it around and doing well that second semester freshman year.

And then I had a bit of a personal tragedy. There was a significant death of a family friend sophomore year, and I didn't have the emotional maturity at the time to cope with that, or to cope with it in a productive way, so I coped with it in maladaptive ways by sort of socializing with friends and putting off my schoolwork. My grades really started to suffer from that, but it was really only second semester of junior year where I really appreciated the damage, and really knew that if I didn't bring it together, that I would have no chance of getting into medical school, which was my goal.

I started seeing a tutor. I started really buckling down and changing my approach, managing my time better, and I ended up doing better senior year but still, I still wasn't nearly competitive enough for medical school. I sort of took those lessons that I learned in managing my situation in undergrad and then transferred it to graduate school, and now I'm actually doing a lot better in graduate school now than I ever did as an undergrad.

And I think that's honestly because I failed so badly in undergrad, because I was able to sort of... I knew the things I did in undergrad, and I was able to do the opposite in graduate school.

> *I typically recommend students avoid discussing academic failures; however, I think this was a little different. It was more than, "I struggled with the MCAT," or "I failed organic chemistry," and instead, "I failed my whole undergraduate career." This also potentially highlights some issues the interviewer may find in the application in terms of poor grades.*

Student B

Student B: I mean, I've had many failures in my life. I would say a time I failed... I mean, when I was in school, when I was in university, college, obviously there were grades that I got that were not good. I got "C"s. I remember in particular, there was one grade I got in organic chemistry at the time. It really crushed me at that time because I knew that that was really going to hurt my chances of... I was already struggling in the sciences, and to get that grade, it was just really... It was really hard. That's when I really was a failure because I know... Even at that time, I knew the implications of that for my prospects for school as far as my GPA.

Dr. Gray: Do you have any non-academic examples?

Student B: Non-academic? Well, the obvious one is applying to medical school, not getting in.

Dr. Gray: That's academic.

Student B: Okay. When I was working in my job, I had a job, I had it for almost 10 years, and I don't know if it's a failure or more of a regret that I feel like I gave too much to the job and I didn't give as much time to my family. I didn't listen to people in my family telling me that I shouldn't spend too much time in the job. I feel like in that sense, I failed, in a way, I would say. I gave too much instead of giving time back into my own life and it hurt me with my family and personally.

> *You can see that the first two answers are academic. Poor grades and not getting into medical school should not be discussed as failures. The last example is more personal, but there's a potential red flag. Medical school will likely be more of a commitment than this student's job. What will their support be once they are in school? What pressure will they have to not study for their exam so they can spend time with family? Students often give me answers that make me question their commitment. Make sure you stay away from that.*

Student C

> *I specifically asked the student about a non-academic failure.*

Student C: I have failed multiple times, many, many times. I think the time that I have failed the worst would be the time that I got very depressed and I did something really bad. I ran my car into my boyfriend's house, and I got arrested. He's my husband now but from that I just learned a very hard lesson in life that the consequence that you pay is unimaginable when you do something that you just don't think clear like that.

> *I love this student's honesty. Unfortunately, this answer raises a lot of red flags. There's always a balance of being true to who you are and telling your story, and making sure you don't incriminate yourself and give the Admissions Committee an easy way to reject you. This type of answer brings up too many questions, so avoid anything like it.*
>
> *This experience was definitely a failure, but it shows more red flags than reflection. It's obvious that this student had*

problems with anger management and other issues, which might make the interviewer reconsider this student for their school. I think we could all picture ourselves getting quite mad, but I would not give that answer in a medical school interview.

In their application, the student would have to talk about their arrest. If you've had something similar, please talk with your lawyer about what you must disclose based on the questions being asked. Try your best to answer the question without raising a ton of red flags, but be able to discuss what you've learned and how you've grown.

Student D

I specifically asked the student about a non-academic failure

Student D: There was a time where I was in a powerlifting competition and I had gone up for my second attempt on a squat and I got it about halfway up but just couldn't make it and it rolled over my head and it actually knocked me out a little bit. Of course, I had to adjust in the acute situation and go back at it and review the video, go over some things with my coach, went back at the third attempt and ended up getting it.

But it was really frustrating that I couldn't reach my full potential because you only get three chances. So, I had to take a step back, reevaluate my squat form, go through really basic drills to get the new form dialed in. That is really frustrating to already be lifting 250 pounds or 275 pounds but now you're working your way back to just doing the bar, but you have to do it the correct way. It's definitely a mindset shift that you have to accept that, hey, I wasn't as good as I could have been. Sometimes you have to take a step back and evaluate where did things go wrong or where can I improve myself?

This student did a good job of telling a story of failing during a competition, then reflecting on that failure and the lessons learned. Obviously, this isn't a dramatic failure, but it's a good example of something you can potentially reflect on and highlight in your journey. Your specific story is important. Your answers don't have to be flashy or dramatic; they just need to be your story.

Why This School?

Student A

Student A: First of all, location. I grew up in the area. I'm familiar with the area. There's data to support a medical student's success if they're sort of close to home. They're… But the mission statement's really what's sort of hooked me into that school, because there's two other schools that are also in the area that are not as high on my list, and it's because they set out from the outset to train and foster empathy within their physicians. And that's the whole game. That's the whole reason to be a doctor, is you got to have empathy with your patients, and I like that it says that on the package.

From the outset, they're like, "We're going to train you to have empathy. We're going to train you to really connect with the patients and really understand their lives. What gets them up in the morning, what motivates them to do things." And I think that's how you render the most effective care. In fact, I don't think that, I know that. That is how you render the most effective care as a physician, is you understand the motivation of your patients. You understand the feelings. That's why that medical school is my top choice.

You'll see that my feedback for this specific question is almost also prefaced with "Keep doing more research into the school. Keep finding those specifics that resonate with you."

In Student A's response, I like the addition of location and the discussion about family support. That said, I do not recommend that location be the first thing you discuss. If you were courting a significant other, and they asked why you wanted to date them, would you lead with, "Well, you live close, so that helps." Not the most flattering answer. The school wants to know that you want to go to the school, not just because it's convenient for you. Bring up location later, after more specific things about the program.

In general, I also do not recommend trying to prove that you know what it's like to be a physician. That is not the goal of this process. "I know the best care is to…" How do you know? You've seen a few physicians, hopefully, through your shadowing, but is that the best care? What most students are trying to do in these situations is say, "Physicians need to have empathy, and I have empathy, too, so you should accept me." Avoid these talking points because you really can't know what it is like to be a physician until you become a physician.

Student B

Student B: The school is first and foremost where I live. It's in my hometown and I want to go to school there to hopefully go to residency there and practice here. It's one of the top schools in the country looking at the rankings. Those are the main reasons why I would like to go there.

Dr. Gray: Do you have any other specifics about the school? Things that resonate with you?

Student B: It has a very strong academic reputation.

Dr. Gray: You said that already. It's one of the top schools in the country.

Student B: Oh, I would say since even when I was in university, they hold a yearly premed conference, at the time, it was for minority students. I think it's still for minority students and the fact that they held this conference every year for minority students—to me it showed that they cared, that they want minorities to succeed and to enter the school. I appreciate that as a minority myself, so I like that about them.

The beginning of this answer was very brief and superficial. The student mentions location and school reputation. Going back to my analogy of courting someone, those aren't going to be very flattering answers. They also aren't specific enough to answer the question. Ideally, you should focus on something very particular, like the school's curriculum, and relate it to you and why you think it will work well for you. Hopefully, you can emphasize a certain program at the school and talk about a similar program you did as an undergrad. The goal of these answers isn't just to list what you read about the school but also to relate them to you.

Student C

Student C: I really liked that this school, in particular, has physical therapists and they have a consortium that they all come to and evaluate cases and figure out what you can learn from each other. I was actually discussing it with one of the doctors that I scribed with and he pointed out something that he learned in his residency from a veterinary medicine student that they had brought on about how in the veterinary medicine world, if a mother is not bonding with their children, they give the mother oxytocin whereas whenever we have mothers with maternal depression, we give antidepressants. So, it's interesting that whenever we give oxytocin, we see the same bonding and maternal support and child mother relationship growth that they see in the veterinary medicine world. I'm really excited to see what else all of these other aspects can bring at this school.

Then honestly, a big benefit to this school in particular is that it's in a nice suburban neighborhood so it's going to be supportive of my family. My husband's going to be able to work well here and I can literally live five minutes from the school and have my kids in the school system here and integrate into the community, which I'm excited about as well.

> *At first glance, I didn't like the answer because it was confusing. I didn't understand the tangent the student went on. Reflecting on it more, I can see why they chose to discuss veterinary medicine, but I think there is a missed opportunity here to focus the answer a little better. What they were talking about was interdisciplinary education. Many medical schools will have physical therapy students, physician assistant students, and other healthcare students taking the same courses in the same buildings, which allows for diversity in thought. If the student focused more on this and less on the medication side of their discussion, it would have been stronger. Many students discuss medications because they think this will make them seem smarter. In this response, it was confusing. You can also see the student mention location at the end of their answer, which is great.*

Student D

Student D: The reason why I really want to go to this school is because from what I've seen... For me I know the physician that I want to be, and ultimately what I aspire to be, and how I want to be able to bridge the gap for a lot of patients who are hopeless and vulnerable. To me I want to be able to integrate myself into a school that would grant me the privilege to care for different patients, as far as an urban academic center for example. Where I can care for a diverse array of patients, as well as still be involved in areas that might be underserved or underrepresented.

Basically, I want to go to this school because for one, the commitment to patients, patient care as far as locally and globally, specifically with student run clinics, the student outreach clinic that you guys have here. A lot of medical schools have student outreach clinics that are built for the uninsured but particularly here, the reason why I'm interested in this one, is because of the interplay of the multiple professions that are involved. From the medical students, and nursing students, and pharmacy students all working together to really provide that care and continuity of it.

But then also the other social aspects of it. The social context of the health, such as physical therapy, psychologists also being involved, as well as legal services to all these students being involved. Really trying to not only provide the care that the patient might need and might not get because they don't have access to it with being uninsured. But also, all the other aspects of the social services that could affect their health.

I think that's really unique about this student outreach clinic that I don't see anywhere else. That's something that I'm really passionate about because I, myself, come from an underrepresented, underserved background. I could be able to identify with that patient population.

But also, the curriculum here, through my pre-clinicals and clinical years, makes sense to me. The phase I, phase II, phase III. Phase I being all the sub-cellular to the organ tissue-based learning. Then coupled with the clinical foundations that you get to be able to do with the patients since day one. Specifically, the one thing that draws me the most about that is that I can also apply, and opt-out, for a medical Spanish course where I learn medical Spanish and be able to work with

Spanish speaking patients for my OSCEs. That to me is something that I'm really passionate about and I feel like I don't get anywhere else.

Lastly, the sense of community, and the culture, and support that you guys have. The ability for this school to really… That it's really receptive to the feedback that students get every year and implements it. The support services that we have for us to succeed and the mentorship. The mentorship, unofficially through the students, when I'm paired up with the MS2, MS3 is a big brother/big sister. Then also the official mentorship program through the advising office. Where I have a mentor specialty or someone that I can identify with that's mentoring me every semester, and ultimately allows me to build a relationship with somebody, and I hope that one day I can be able to be that mentor for somebody else as they progress.

> *On the face of it, you may think this is a great, in-depth answer. Unfortunately, a lot of it is very generic—at least in the way the student presented it. The student led with urban, academic medicine. A majority of medical schools in this country are located in urban locations that give students access to a diverse patient population. Most, if not all, medical schools have free clinics for students.*
>
> *Instead of painting a picture of the school with broad strokes, narrow it down to specifics like naming the different programs that resonate with you and then explain why they resonate with you.*

Student E

Student E: After moving around, I really recognized that the place you grew up and the communities we come from really have a lot more impact than I thought it would. And so, staying local is attractive to me. But more importantly, I've seen that this school has a really great problem-based learning program and I've really felt that that's a really amazing learning environment. I've spoken with a couple of students who have really had a great impression of that system, so that's super attractive to me. The focus to really keep people in this state, I thought was really incredible. For me, it's not as much of a, "Hey, I have a better chance of admission," but overall that they're really focusing on the community, which is huge. I've been involved with some efforts rebuilding community there, and so keeping things local is super important. And then anything else beyond that is having really great, strong LGBT programs are important for me. I transitioned over the last few years, and knowing that a school is accepting is important. You have multiple different LGBT programs, even within the school of medicine.

> *I think the student did a great job with this answer but in the wrong order. I would have focused on the LGBT programs first because that seems like it's the most personal for the student. The student led, again, with location, which should go at the end. They mentioned the school's problem-based learning (PBL) curriculum, which is great, but they could have improved their answer by focusing on why it would work well for them, not just that others liked it. What was their exposure to PBL? Have they been in that curriculum before? How did they do? That's how you can tie together specific aspects of the school to who you are and make your answer stronger.*

Should We Have an Opt-out Organ Donation System?

Student A

Student A: Yes, I agree. The opt-out is a bit like how we do vaccinations now, where instead of saying, "Would you like to be an organ donor," you automatically make them an organ donor. And this is typically what I associate with getting your driver's license. They do this sort of thing in Europe, and it's really helped the organ shortages over there. I believe they started a program there in the early 2000s in Spain, and it's really helped with an organ shortage that they were having. And I really believe that that would help a lot with a lot of the issues we have in the United States about procuring organs for donation. Go up to the DMV. They ask you, "Would you like to be an organ donor?" And instead, they'd say, "Would you like to opt-out of organ donation?" Otherwise, you'd automatically be entered into the program.

Dr. Gray: Why do you think that's such a powerful difference in the numbers of people that actually donate organs?

Student A: Oh, because it's operating in a negative, right? You're not actually asking someone to do something. Just in my own personal experience, it's a lot easier to... it's a lot easier to say, "Yes" to something. Or it's a lot harder to say, "Yes" to something. Right?

You're asking someone, "Would you like to be an organ donor?" That's kind of hard to do. You're kind of having to put a little bit of effort into that versus, "Oh, I'm already there. Oh, okay, since I'm already entered let's not bother. No big deal. Just keep me in."

> *This student was well aware of the opt-out versus opt-in organ donation sign-up differences. They do a great job giving their opinion right away, which I think is important for moral and ethical questions; then they support their opinion with their thought process and information from other places that are doing something similar. This student also did well on the insurance question, and I asked how they stay informed. They mentioned listening to podcasts, specifically The Daily Zeitgeist.*
>
> *Remember that for these moral and ethical questions, your goal isn't to give the "right" answer but rather to provide an answer that fits your morals and ethics. Then, support that decision with your thought process and other information, including any anecdotes from your life.*

Student B

Student B: Yes, because of maybe religious reasons or personal reasons. There's some individuals that don't believe in that or that may be an ethical issue for them. So, people should have the right to opt-out if they choose. That's my personal belief.

Dr. Gray: Well, let me rephrase that. Right now, we have an opt-in system, correct?

Student B: Yes, you can sign up.

Dr. Gray: Yeah. So right now, you have to say, yes, I want to be an organ donor. In an opt-out system you would be forced to say no, I don't want to be an organ donor.

Student B: Right. So, I think that if people want to opt-out to not be an organ donor, I believe people should have the right to do that. Yes.

> *You can see I struggled with this student because I wasn't sure they understood the question because of the brief response. I tried to rephrase and was met with another brief response, which was only that they thought people should be able to opt-out. Supporting your answer with your thought process is a must. These types of questions are not yes or no questions. Do your best to expand and show your understanding. Talk about where we are right now and where we may be going based on the question.*
>
> *If, based on your own religious beliefs, you want to answer a question a certain way, you can and should do that. Remember, there are no right answers. The interviewer wants to learn who you are, including your personal beliefs, which are relevant and can help strengthen your answer. If you're not comfortable doing that, then don't. But if you are, then I think you should, while continuing to expand and show an understanding of the topic.*

Student C

Student C: I don't think we should because to donate an organ, I believe we have to sign a consent form when we… I don't know about other states, but in state of Texas when we provide driver license, we actually have the way to just say that we want to donate our organ or not. So that's the decision.

Dr. Gray: That's an opt-in system. So, the opt-out system would be when you go and get your driver's license, you say, "No thank you, I don't want to be an organ donor." Instead of saying, "Yes, I want to be an organ donor."

Student C: Yes. If that's the case, then yes, the opt-out option should be there because you got to give a person the choice that they want to make. You can't really force the person to do what they want to do or what they don't want to do.

> *You can see from the answer, and how brief it is, that this student didn't understand opt-out versus opt-in. I wanted to give you this*

example because if you don't fully understand the question, you should let the interviewer know. Tell them you're not sure what opt-out means and ask if they can explain it to you. As soon as I did that, the student understood and changed their answer. Your interviewer may not redirect you as I did here. Again, this answer was pretty superficial, but I'm not surprised because of the lack of understanding in the first place.

Remember that your goal is not to know everything but to be able to discuss anything. Based on your own upbringing, morals, and ethics, you should be able to discuss any topic, even if you're not completely aware of the situation. Make it known, while answering, that you're not knowledgeable about the topic, but keep talking and discussing.

Student D

Student D: I would say yes. In that people have differing religious views that may not coincide with the thought process behind organ transplant or organ donation. I do believe that other circumstances involved with the emotions of families when they're dealing with the loved ones that are giving those organs to those in need also play a large role in organ donation.

You can see here, again, that the student doesn't really do a great job of answering the question. The student also brings in irrelevant information—the discussion of family isn't part of the opt-out versus opt-in system. When a student is not confident in the topic, this is the typical answer given to the interviewer. Make sure, as you are preparing for your interviews, that you do enough research to have some understanding of how things work in this country, but also be confident enough to say "I don't know" when presented with a topic with which you are not familiar.

Should We Have Medicare for All?

Student A

Student A: Oh, a Medicare for All type system. Okay. I think that we definitely should, and I think that would go a long way to increase accessibility. Now, increase accessibility, increase the affordability of the system.

Now, there's a couple of ways that we could go about doing this. I think that, for one, people need to realize that using taxes to pay into that sort of system, whether it's an English type system where all the hospitals are government run, and all the hospital employees, the doctors, the nurses, all the staff are government employees, or if it's like a German or a French type system where it's a private hospital and the government just sort of pays into it. I think that that system is a little bit better just because I think it offers a little bit more autonomy to each hospital and sort of run how they feel it needs to be run.

But I think that the first step is getting people to actually realize that it's cheaper, because paying into insurance now for like a private plan through employment would actually be more expensive than using taxes to pay for sort of a more universal healthcare system. That's it.

Dr. Gray: How do we educate people that it is cheaper?

Student A: Oh, that don't want to pay? That's a really tough question, honestly, and that's, I think, a little bit of winning the hearts and minds. I think it's more on the politicians to convince people to pay in the first place, and so there has to be quite a bit of front-end loading.

I'm thinking about in... when the Obamacare legislation was passed, I think in 2012, there was a whole lot of backlash towards it. There was a lot of backlash leading up to it about how it would ruin healthcare, about how it would make it so much more expensive. And then, in 2016 when there, there was another concerted campaign to repeal it when our current president was campaigning upon repealing it, there was a massive backlash, and people who had previously opposed the legislation actually came around to benefit a lot from it and to support it.

Ideally, people wouldn't have that thought, but the people that do would... It'd be like taxes, I suppose. You get arrested for not paying your taxes, or rather, you get in trouble for not paying your taxes, so I think it would be a similar sort of situation.

> *The student did an amazing job with this question. They showed an understanding of our system as well as different healthcare systems around the world. The student talked about their stance and did a good job of demonstrating the thought process behind it. Remember, you don't have to have this much understanding of the different healthcare systems to answer this question well—you just need to give your thoughts. If you don't have a deeper understanding, like this student, your answer could be even stronger by expanding on your opinion and the thought process behind it.*

Student B

Student B: I do believe in Medicare for All. I think it's a viable alternative to what we have now. The healthcare system in this country is not good. It's broken, and I believe that it needs to be changed, and Medicare for All is a good option to that.

> *This student does not really answer the question. When asked why the answer was short and not supported by anything, they mentioned they thought the answers had to be very quick. The student sacrificed answering the question and supporting it with their thought process because they were unaware of normal interview etiquette. That's okay for a mock interview, like this, because now they know better, and so do you. You need to answer the question. You obviously don't want to talk for 30 minutes when you answer, but your response needs to be long enough to give your thoughts and support your decision.*

Student C

Student C: I think we should. I do not really know that well about the Medicare and Medicaid system. I fail again.

Even though this student gave up on the answer during the mock interview, I wanted to put it in the book because this could happen to you. You may get a question that you don't know anything about; it's okay to admit you don't know and ask the interviewer to give you some background information to help you answer the question. Asking for clarification and more information is not failing. Giving up is failing—as this student did.

I would recommend reading The Healthcare Handbook *to give you some deeper insight into the healthcare industry.*

Student D

Student D: I think ethically, yes, because I think that everybody deserves quality health care, but do I think that it's possible, at least at this state and time? Not necessarily. I like the idea of everybody deserves it. It is a right, in my mind, but I understand that the system that we already have right now would need a lot of changes to get there as well as culturally we would need a lot of changes to get that acceptance and support within the people as well.

Dr. Gray: Do you think it would be more expensive or less expensive for people to have a Medicare for All system?

Student: I think initially it is going to take a higher cost just to get the programs running, to get new infrastructure set up. Of course, we're going to be taking a lot of new patients and a lot of new care, but I believe in the long run the preventative costs will outweigh that and eventually we will break even and end up better off for it.

The student did a good job looking forward and talking about what they think we should have while also talking about the current situation and why we aren't getting there. I think the response could have been made a little stronger by including more background knowledge or bringing in some understanding of other country's healthcare systems.

Student E

Student E: Yes. I would say yes to that, 100%. Having been in a career where I'm paying into private insurance, I see that there are a lot of holes in insurance, and insurance billing, and how insurance works for the patient, and the stress it puts on a lot of people financially. I don't think Medicare should be free. I think there should be a cost efficiency type of working mechanism, where you pay what you can, but I do think that healthcare should be available to all for... Or with an affordable... Making it affordable for everyone.

Dr. Gray: You think that paying should be above and beyond taxes to support it?

Student E: I would say yes it goes way beyond taxes. In that, like I said before, paying what you can and taking into account income, and then other circumstances regarding income that has to do more with social services, and I guess census even, and what your family makes, or what you make, or what an individual makes to sustain their lives while also having access to healthcare.

Dr. Gray: Why not just build that into the tax system because that's how taxes are setup now—people pay what they can afford. Right? Taxes are based on income.

Student E: Again, I mean that's just... Taxes take a lot out of people's income, depending on whatever tax bracket you fall into. So, it's not always a measure of someone's ability to pay for healthcare. For instance, the average person, where I live, making less than $40,000 a year—they're paying upwards of $600, $700 per month in taxes to the federal and local government. So, it's not necessarily a measure of what they're able to pay. Those other social services and other measures of someone's inability or ability to pay for healthcare need to be taken into account as well.

This student did a good job discussing their thoughts on Medicare for All and bringing in some personal perspective, both from being a nontraditional student, having a career and needing health insurance, and talking about ways to make it more affordable for the government. As I've mentioned previously, bringing in other knowledge—current plans to change our healthcare system, or healthcare systems in other countries—is a way to expand your discussion and show that you've done your research. This is a good example of an answer that I personally didn't understand, but it was what the student believed. I could have dug in deeper to try to understand more, but I was comfortable with the outcome.

A very common concern with these types of questions is how political they can get. I recommend you keep politics out of your answer, but sometimes you can't, and you shouldn't necessarily make that your goal. Remember, your goal is to be you and communicate your thoughts and beliefs, and sometimes that is based on your political preferences. What you don't want to do is to be polarizing. You don't want to say, "All conservatives are idiots," or, "All liberals are idiots." That's never the answer.

Student F

Student F: I think that we need something definitely different than what we have now. I'm not sure if Medicaid for All is the correct answer. I don't know that we've really found a system that would work for everyone. Mostly, cost wise, and trying to figure out what's considered a tax and what's not. I know that that's a big argument with it, and I haven't really dove into that a whole lot. I know from Medicaid, when my children were on Medicaid, it was very limited. I don't know if Medicare for All would be like that, where they would be... I felt like they weren't given the care that they needed in a timely manner. It was really hard to find physicians that would do certain procedures or would see them besides certain time blocks, and I don't know if there would still be a market for private insurance if someone just wasn't happy with what was available from Medicare for All.

I also talked to my friends in Canada about their system, and they can see emergency medicine fairly easy, they can see their primary care fairly easy, but they have told me that it's really hard to get into specialists because the specialists, at least in their experiences, from what they've shared with me, they've got a shortage of specialists because they don't get paid what they used to, or what our specialists would get paid here in the States.

And so, it's not as big of a push, I guess, for specialists, at least in their areas. So, I would worry about that being an effect. Other than that, I don't really have a whole lot of experience digging into the details.

> *Here, the student did a good job talking about personal experiences, as well as bringing in a discussion with a friend about the Canadian healthcare system. This was a longer answer, possibly because of a lack of confidence in their answer. You can't really see that in this transcript, but we talked about it afterward. It's a very common strategy that students use when they lack confidence in their understanding—they keep talking until they find something that works.*
>
> *It's frequent for students to talk about wait times in Canada and other universal or single-payer healthcare systems. What they fail to realize is that we have the same wait issues for specialists, even within our current healthcare system. It's less a function of the specialization of medicine and more a function of how that healthcare is being paid.*

Student G

Student G: Overwhelmingly, resoundingly yes. I think that Medicare for All would be a great policy to be implemented in the near future. There are so many, I guess, roadblocks that I've found that physicians and physician assistants run into when dealing with patients. Recently, I was at a shadowing experience where a few of the providers were talking about United, and the patients having United. And they said when these United patients come in, man, it's almost like a hospital service, because they can never get out of the hospital. So, I think alleviating that private insurance would in fact, and adopting a Medicare for All system, would in fact be beneficial to the patients and the physicians alike. However, I do understand that Medicare is… Or excuse me, healthcare is expensive, and I think we really need to think hard about how that's going to get paid for, of course.

> *This answer seemed to be okay on the surface, but when you look at the anecdote, it was a little confusing. The discussion about United, the healthcare insurance company, left me confused as to what the*

student was actually talking about. It wasn't tied to how private insurance was an issue. At the end, the student brought up paying for Medicare for All. Whenever you bring up an issue, it's a good opportunity to mention potential solutions. They could have followed up with, "We really need to think hard" and "Here are some of my thoughts."

Student H

Student H: Absolutely. I think that of course, first and foremost, that healthcare is a basic human right, and I believe that with the current system we have right now, which is largely a for-profit one, having that middleman of the insurance agencies artificially just inflates costs, and by removing that middleman, we may be able to save costs. And there's many different ways we can implement that in an affordable way, but overall, I think that without transitioning to a Medicare for All program, that we have intense inequalities that really contribute to people not having access to healthcare. It's continuing to proliferate as we allow for that discrepancy between people who have insurance and don't, to continue to raise as it is.

This is a good example of a student who is very supportive of one side of the issue, and they give some good thoughts to defend their answer. The answer could be stronger and more complete with a little bit of the counterargument as well. Often referred to as "giving both sides of the argument," the student could have mentioned why people don't want to have a Medicare for All system, or what they perceive as some of the big obstacles to implementing it.

What is Your Greatest Strength?

Student A

Student A: I think my greatest strength is my enthusiasm. I am a definitely a both feet kind of guy. After I graduated college in 2017, I was kind of lazing around a little bit during the summer and sort of dawdling around looking for jobs. And finally, I was like, "You know what, I'm not getting a job in my field," which was medicine or research. I was looking for jobs in sort of both areas and no one was biting, so I was like, "You know what, I'm just going to send out a bunch of applications to a bunch of local businesses in my hometown, and we'll see what happens."

I ended up getting two callbacks at two different places, so I ended up working 60-hour weeks accepting both jobs, working as a prep cook and as a sort of a customer support at a plant nursery. And then once my job got ... Once I actually got hired by a university to do some research, it was in Phoenix, Arizona, and I was in Dallas, so I moved out to Phoenix, and I started, basically, immediately doing research as the project lead for this massive interdisciplinary project. I think that's my greatest strength is like, enthusiasm. I really go in and attack something head on.

> *This answer has some good parts and some pieces that could be improved. I like how the student used examples to highlight the point they were trying to make. Because the answer was a little long and not completely straightforward, I was a little confused as to where the student was going. I'm also not sure if the example given shows enthusiasm or dedication. I frequently hear an answer to this question and then have to let the student know that their example didn't illustrate their stated strength. Be careful with that.*

Student B

Student B: I believe my greatest strength is that I'm a very determined individual. I work hard, and I… When I have a task in front of me, I work hard to achieve it no matter what the obstacles in my way. I don't like to take, "No" for an answer. I just keep going until I achieve it, especially if it's something that I want to achieve. I don't give up on what I want to achieve.

Dr. Gray: Do you have a specific example to support that?

Student B: Well, I think the number one example is trying to enter medical school. I graduated from university back in 2003. It's 2020. I'm still here. I'm trying to enter medical school. Of course, I've done other things in my life since that time, but it's something…This dream of mine to become a doctor is something that I never gave up on, and it's something that I want to accomplish, and I hopefully will accomplish. That's where I would say my best example of that is.

> *An answer without an example is almost always going to be cliché. Not taking "no" for an answer, without an instance of what that looks like for you, doesn't tell the interviewer anything. As best as you can, give an anecdote to support your answer.*
>
> *Just as I recommend avoiding academic examples for questions about failure, I wouldn't use examples of not getting into medical school and reapplying to show determination. Look for deeper examples that show who you are.*
>
> *There was one small red flag in this answer that I discussed with the student afterward. Saying you've wanted to be a doctor for 17 years concerns me. Either you're really not dedicated to it, you're delusional, or something else. Something just doesn't add up. Make sure you're not giving the interviewer more questions than answers.*

Student C

Student C: I think that I'm very organized and have a great attention to detail. That's probably one of my strengths that has served me very well in my academic journey so far.

Dr. Gray: Do you have a specific example?

Student C: In my group projects and stuff like that I usually be able to spot the mistake that a lot of people make and improve that way. A lot of time people don't really, when they read the project description, they don't read word by word and when they finish the project, they have a lot of things that they miss when it's already stated in the project description. So, because of my attention to detail, I kind of avoid those small mistakes that actually matters a lot.

> *Here's another example of a student giving an answer without any supportive evidence—an anecdote. When prompted for one, they gave a story in which they decided to throw their classmates under*

the bus. They didn't need to call out their classmates' lack of attention to detail to highlight their own attention to detail. Don't compare yourself to anyone else. Focus on you, and you alone.

Student D

Student D: I think my ability to plan and think ahead. I have a lot going on in my life and I recognize that, but the way that I'm able to handle that is to plan and prioritize and make sure that the more important things are getting focused on and I know how to say no when I need to.

Dr. Gray: Do you have an example of that?

Student D: For example, whenever I was studying for the MCAT, I was also trying to peak for a national powerlifting competition. But I recognized that my MCAT studies needed to take more priority. I was still homeschooling my own kids, so I still had mom responsibilities and my MCAT responsibilities and I had to let powerlifting go for a bit and let it slide. Then once I was done with my MCAT, I was able to come back to it, had that open free time. So, I recognized that life can come in phases and so sometimes a priority is going to be greater in one phase and then a different priority will rise up in a different phase.

This is a great example of turning a generic "I'm good at planning" answer with no example into a very strong answer that highlights everything the student has been able to accomplish with their other responsibilities. This shows me hard work, dedication, motivation, and other amazing intangibles that they'll add to the class.

Student E

Student E: I think my greatest strength is definitely my perseverance and that any obstacle I face I'm able to tackle it, and set myself above the rest, in that when I set out for a goal, I know I'm going to accomplish that goal given any circumstances surrounding said goal. For instance, being a single mom, and going to school, and also working full-time. That being my hierarchy with my family being first, school being second, and then my work life being last. With that, whether it be grades interfering with goals or my work schedule, I'm able to maintain a balance that helps me get through said obstacles.

Dr. Gray: Do you have a specific example of an obstacle that you've had to overcome? Something that shows your perseverance?

Student E: Yes, definitely. I'm dealing with childcare issues that's impacting my school schedule. That started two semesters ago. I've since fixed that situation but within that I lost my childcare and my grades kind of slipped. For instance, I took orgo and I took calculus II, and got Ds in both classes. The semester after I was able to remedy my childcare situation, work on what I could do with what I was given and having to retake said classes, and I got "A"s the following semester, so fall 2019.

> *Once probed for an example, the student was able to solidify their original response to the question. You may think the examples they gave originally were good enough, but when you examine them, they are generic. Being a single mom, working, and going to school are not the example—those are just the setting for the example given after being prompted.*
>
> *One thing that stands out as something to avoid is the comparison made early on: "Set myself above the rest." Do not try to prove your superiority over others during this process—both in your applications and at your interviews.*

Student F

Student F: I think my greatest strength would potentially be my… I would say probably… in a modest way I would say probably my perseverance. I find that all my life I've been facing resistance, or some type of adversity, or something that would challenge me to be in a situation where I could have easily said, "Okay, well this is the cards that life dealt me," or, "This is the situation that I'm in, so now I got to just take this loss."

Specifically, like in high school, I knew that I was not really meant to go to college because that's not what kids from my high school did, but I still worked really hard to make that happen. Because then I wanted to get an education and get out of the life that I was in. When I got to college, I had advisors telling me that I wouldn't get into the biomedical engineering program because my GPA was too low or I wouldn't be able to go to medical school because candidates with better GPAs, 3.8s, weren't even getting into medical school. Even though they're probably in good nature just trying to look out for me, trying to help me in the best they can, I still went against the odds to try to persevere. I began to be able to make the life that I wanted.

I feel like there's always things that present themselves to box you in or prevent you from going certain places, or maybe temptations that can easily make you comfortable, but I always persevere to things that I truly am passionate about… Who I am and who I want to become.

I think the word is perseverance for that, but I keep going or grit. Yeah, I think that would probably be my greatest strength but yeah.

> *This is a good example of a student giving an answer and then following it up with a supporting story. It's a little long, but the student did a good job of highlighting their journey, including overcoming a lot of obstacles. The one part I might have left out is the "negative" side of an advisor telling them they couldn't get into medical school. A lot of students try to bring in a story like this to show perseverance, but it is unconstructive and can be avoided.*

Student G

Student G: Probably resilience and determination. I would go with those.

Dr. Gray: Would you care to expand?

Student G: Sure. I guess because I've gone through so much in life, a lot of obstacles thrown my way, a lot of things trying to deter me from my path, just things knocking me down. I've always brushed it off, gotten back up, and reassessed my goals, my path, and just determined a new way to get to where I want to go.

> *This is another example of how students can fail to develop and support their answers. When prompted to expand, they gave*

definitions of resilience and determination, but didn't give examples of resilience and determination in their own life. Hopefully, by now, you can see the difference that a good anecdote from your life can make in your answer.

Why Are You Switching to Medicine? (For Nontrads)

Student A

Dr. Gray: So, you're a nurse now, and so why make the switch to medicine? Obviously, the increased debt, the time away from making money, the training time to become a physician, why switch careers at this point?

Student A: Well, nursing was actually my plan B. I had wanted to become a physician right out of high school, and had applied for school, couldn't afford it, and that's the point where life kind of happened and got in the way. I got into a relationship, and he was abusive. Kept me away from my dreams, and I finally realized I had to do something to get out of that situation. So, I signed up for nursing school, knowing that, as a nurse, I could afford to take care of my kids on my own and get away from that.

But I also majored in biology while I was in nursing school, and took some extra classes just knowing that, at some point, I wanted to go back and try again as premed. And so now that my children are older, I've reevaluated some things. We actually went to one of our new physician appointments after I got a new job and had to switch to a different hospital system with my doctors. And she was talking to my daughter and I about medicine, and how it would be for a non-traditional student to try to go back for premed and to get into medical school.

And it was just very encouraging, and the more I thought about it, the more I'm like, "You know, my kids are young adults now. This would be the time for me to try to go back to it." And so, I looked into it a little bit more, and realized I wasn't that far off as far as prerequisites go, and so I signed up for school. I had three days before classes started that semester, and I went ahead and signed up, and dug into it a little bit deeper, and realized that, yeah, that is where I wanted to be.

I've never really been satisfied as a nurse. It's definitely saved me from a lot of bad situations that could've happened as a single parent, and it served me very well, but I've just never been completely satisfied.

The student had a good story but ultimately didn't answer the question. I wanted to include this example because it's very common for students to fail to answer the question, especially when diving into a story. Make sure that when you begin your answer, you are keeping track of the question and where you want to go with your response to answer the question. This answer was really just, "I was premed to begin with, and I talked to a physician, and it sounds like now is a good time to try it."

For nontraditional students, it's very important to focus on "why medicine" and not just "why not [insert career here]." The answer was more focused on "I've never really been satisfied as a nurse" and how it was an escape from a bad situation. This doesn't tell me that they should be a physician. Make sure you're painting that picture of "why medicine" and "why now."

What Do You Think About the Right to Die or Death with Dignity Laws?

Student A

Student A: You know, physicians kind of have the principle of "do no harm," and that kind of goes against it, I would say. So, while we do have to consider the patients' wishes, if they come in and seek medical care, I think it's our duty to educate the patients on kind of how we feel about that, and I guess provide our thoughts and opinions on how they should go about treatment and seeking end-of-life care. I think all of the options should definitely be laid in front of them, but ultimately, I do support patients' autonomy and I do support their decision in right to die.

This example demonstrates the importance of making sure the interviewer knows your stance before you continue with your thought process. At the start, it didn't sound like this student supported the right to die, but as the discussion went on, they came to that conclusion. I'm not sure if the student came to this position after starting to talk, or if they knew they were going there all along, but it would have been better to state the opinion first.

SECTION III

OUTCOMES

WAITLISTED

After your interview, there are typically three responses from the school: accepted, rejected, and waitlisted. Being waitlisted can be a huge blow to your confidence. You left the interview thinking you nailed it—you told your friends and family you had an amazing time, and you hope to get an acceptance to that school. You think you will get in because you had a great day and connected well with the interviewers.

Sometimes, though, despite how well your interviews went, you still may not get an acceptance. Every school is a little bit different in how they review their students with the Admissions Committee. Some schools will ignore everything in your application other than your interview. Others will take your interview and all of the other information in your application and compare that to other students. Some schools may only be interviewing for waitlist spots, depending on when you are interviewing during the application cycle. Some schools may waitlist almost everyone until later in the application cycle when they make their final decisions.

Just know that a waitlist doesn't mean *no*. A waitlist means, "We like you, but we don't have room for you," or, "We like you, but we're not sure how much yet." It can also mean, "We're not sure how much we like you, but we don't hate you, so you're not going to get rejected right away." No matter the reason, getting waitlisted can be very frustrating. You typically have to wait a very long time, especially if that school is your only interview, to know whether or not you're going to get into medical school or if you'll need to reapply.

I love seeing success stories online of a student who is in the middle of getting their applications ready for the next cycle, and they finally receive their acceptance.

Next Steps

What do you do after you are waitlisted? I recommend you thank the school for the waitlist. It may seem weird to say, "Thank you very much for waitlisting me," but you can use it as another piece of communication with the school. They are communicating with you about your application, so you should communicate back to them to let them know you appreciate still being considered, and you are still very interested in going to their school, and you look forward to hearing from them in the future.

Unfortunately, not every school is very waitlist friendly. Some schools will rank their waitlist and will tell you where you are on that list. Many schools don't rank their waitlist, but they review every student on their waitlist when they have an available seat. Those schools will likely not tell you anything about their process or your position on the list.

Updating the Schools

If you have new information that you think would be looked at favorably after you are waitlisted, be very careful before you start rushing to tell every school that new information. Make sure that during this time, you are abiding by their communication rules. Some schools don't want any communication from you. Some schools will only accept updates through a specific channel, like a web portal. This is information that is typically given when you interview. You really have to pay attention to each school's rules to know whether or not you should communicate with the school outside of saying, "Thank you for the waitlist."

Waitlist Movement

Waitlist movement is the term used to discuss when people are being removed from the waitlist and accepted to medical school. There is typically a lot of movement near the end of the application cycle as students are required to narrow down their acceptances to one school.

For example, a student who has four acceptances will eventually need to withdraw their acceptances from three other schools. If you are this student, please withdraw your acceptance as soon as you know you will not be going to a certain school. This will allow the school to extend an acceptance to another student.

For AMCAS, this is recommended around the end of April (search for "AMCAS traffic rules" online). That said, when a student withdraws an acceptance from a school, this does not always open up a "real seat" for someone else to take. The reason is that every medical school typically extends more offers than they can actually accept because there will always be a percentage of students who are accepted who don't attend because they are accepted elsewhere.

Every year, from the end of April to the beginning of May, I receive a lot of emails from students who were waitlisted and who suddenly start to get those messages and phone calls from Admissions Committees letting them know they have been taken off the waitlist and accepted.

The application process is long. Waiting is painful, but a waitlist does not mean a no, so continue to improve your application, stay involved, stay positive, and, as much as you can, continue thinking about potential next steps.

If you are not accepted off of a waitlist, read the chapter about rejection and reapplying.

ACCEPTED, NOW WHAT?

Congratulations, you've been accepted! Now what? That's the biggest question that most students have after they've been accepted. What do you do? Let me first start off by saying that you don't have to do anything. Once you start medical school, your life is going to change forever. Not for the worse, not for the better—it's just going to change. There will be a new norm that you will settle into.

When you start medical school, you'll be taking classes that you may have taken before—but at a whole new level. There is nothing that you can do that will help you to prepare for the intensity of medical school classes. You can try to pre-read, or take an anatomy class, but ultimately nothing that you do can truly prepare you for medical school.

The biggest piece of advice that most medical students give is that once you are accepted, you should go do something to celebrate your acceptance. Travel, if you can afford it. Take a vacation and go somewhere that you've always wanted to go but couldn't because you were too busy with your head down in the books or preparing for the MCAT. If you can't afford a vacation, that's okay—take a staycation. Just relax. Do what you need to do to pay the bills, pay off your credit cards from application season, or start saving for medical school, but please don't try to prepare for medical school classes.

Prereqs

If you haven't finished all of your prereqs, you'll need to make sure you complete them before you start medical school. Double and triple check with the school to make sure they don't have a random required class that you didn't see before. One of the worst things that can happen is not finishing something that is required for matriculation and having your acceptance withdrawn.

You also have to make sure, even though you are accepted, that you stay on top of your grades. If you think that just because you're accepted, you can get away with failing the last set of classes, that is not true. If that happens, medical schools can withdraw your acceptance.

Paperwork

After you've been accepted, there is a lot of paperwork that will come your way. Make sure you stay organized and stay on top of everything.

The absolute first thing you need to make sure you do is to accept the acceptance and put down the deposit to hold your seat. Can you imagine getting one acceptance to medical school, only to throw it away because you failed to let the school know you wanted to go?

You will also likely need to do some healthcare-related things—like getting fully immunized if you have not already.

Most schools will send you paperwork for background checks, financing, accommodations, and more. For schools with multiple campuses or different learning tracks, you may need to make those selections at this time, too. Some schools have you make those selections on your interview day or during the secondary process.

How to Handle Multiple Acceptances

What happens if you are lucky enough to receive multiple acceptances to medical school? The first thing you should do is one of the most basic things that everyone recommends when it comes to making decisions—a pros and cons list. Take a piece of paper, fold it in half, draw a line down the middle, write "Pros" on one side and "Cons" on the other, and the school name at the top. Do this for each school where you have been accepted.

What are the pros of going to that school? Does that school have the research that you want or easy access to a residency you're interested in? Is there a mentor with whom you are excited to work? Are friends from college accepted there as well? Is a loved one accepted? Are there any other potential reasons that you see as "pros" like curriculum, class size, weather, or location?

On the other side, write down the cons. Is the class size too big? Is the weather too cold? Is the location too far? Is tuition too expensive? Do they not have a department for the specialty you are interested in? Are there any other variables you are concerned about that the school falls short on?

Ultimately, what you have to know is that any medical school is going to prepare you well enough to be an amazing physician in the future. Of course, you are the one who has to put in the hard work and dedication to be a great physician, or else no matter what school you go to, including Harvard or WashU, you will not succeed. You have to want it.

Increased Access

I'm a firm believer in networking. Where you go to school can have a direct impact on the network that you can build. You still have to put in the work to build that network, and you have to be someone with whom others will want to network, but having someone with whom you can network on the same campus will be easier than doing it through email. Think through the network that each school can potentially open up for you.

I do not think the network of the medical school should be the biggest variable in your decision—just one of many. I do think the network you create during residency is potentially more important than the one you will build in medical school. I don't want to put too much weight into networks in medical school, but it is something to consider.

Financial Aid

The financial impact of attending one school versus another should be something you think about as well. I don't think it is as easy as saying you should go to the cheapest school. Again, it is just one more variable to consider.

If you have two acceptances, one of the schools may give you financial aid, while the other one may not. In this situation, it is completely acceptable to reach out to the school that has not given you financial aid and ask for it. That said, you have to want to attend the school where you are requesting money. Don't make it a game and start pitting the schools against each other to see who will give you the most money. You want to be respectful of their time and resources as you are making your decision.

You should call them (or email—whatever their communication preference) and honestly tell them, "I really want to go to your school, but another school has given me this financial aid package. Is there anything you can do to make my decision to come to your school less stressful financially?"

There are some schools out there, like NYU and WashU, and probably many others after this book was written, that are offering free tuition. If you get into one of those schools, I think it would be a pretty easy decision. Not needing to take out loans for tuition will make it easier to avoid making decisions based on the financial impact of your medical school loans. If you have two schools that have accepted you with free tuition, then you're back in the same boat of making the pros and cons list to figure out where you want to go.

Trust Your Gut

Ultimately, you need to trust your gut. Recently, I had a student who was accepted to WashU, Vanderbilt, Harvard, University of Virginia, and others. They could easily tell me which ones gave them great vibes and which ones did not. That should definitely play into your decision of where you want to go to medical school. The culture of that school may not fit well with you, and that is okay, even if it is what you consider a top school in the country and one that everyone is pushing you towards. I hear too often from students who struggle in medical school because they went to the wrong one, picking the top-ranked school instead of the school that would have been a better fit for them.

"Remember, don't go to a 'great school.' Go to a school that will make you great."

Second Looks

Many medical schools offer accepted students an opportunity to come back to campus and the surrounding area during a less stressful time. The interview day can be a blur, filled with stress and anxiety, and students need the chance to come back knowing they *will be* a medical student at that school if they choose it.

Second look days are the perfect opportunity to bring other decision-makers as well. If you will be relocating with a significant other, you likely didn't bring them with you for your interview day. The second look day is a great time to bring all those who are involved and supporting you on your journey.

Withdrawing Your Acceptances and Canceling Interviews

As soon as you've settled on one school, help your classmates and future colleagues by removing yourself from every other school where you've been accepted. Also, cancel your future interviews. Doing this will allow medical schools to invite more students to interview and to start accepting students off of their waitlist.

Here is an example of how to notify schools that you are withdrawing your acceptance:

Dear Admissions Committee,

I am grateful for the time your school and committee have given me during this application cycle. I have received an acceptance from another school and therefore would like to withdraw my acceptance from your school.

Regards,
YOUR NAME
AMCAS #12345678

REJECTION AND REAPPLYING

What do you need to do if you get to the end of an application cycle and you have zero acceptances? I remember being in this situation the first time I applied to medical school. I had two interviews, and I was rejected from both of those schools.

In the heat of the moment, I thought the universe was telling me I couldn't be a doctor, and I would never get into medical school. That was just my own insecurities talking, and my perception. The medical schools were just telling me, "Not right now—not this cycle." After I regrouped and recommitted to getting in, I applied again and got in the second time.

When you are applying to medical school, you are trying to do everything to the best of your ability: getting good grades, having a good MCAT score, shadowing, volunteering, attaining clinical experience, all while potentially trying to be a good mom or a good dad, or a good spouse, and trying to put food on the table and a roof over your head. Sometimes it feels like it's just too much, and then when you go through an application cycle and don't get any acceptances after spending thousands of dollars on your applications, you may want to just give up. Many people do, and it's unfortunate.

Let me stop you from doing that. Yes, being rejected from medical school hurts. It's not easy, but it's also not the end. It's only the end if you quit. If you find yourself in this situation, you need to reach out to the schools where you interviewed and ask for feedback. If you did not interview at any schools, I would reach out to every school and ask for feedback.

Most schools won't have the time or resources to give you individualized feedback, but if you don't ask, you won't get it. Remember, medical schools receive thousands upon thousands of applications, and most Admissions Committees are pretty small. Ask nicely and, hopefully, you'll get some valuable comments.

I did an episode of *The Premed Years* with Dr. Leila Amiri, who at the time the Director of Admissions from the University of Illinois, Chicago School of Medicine, about common issues that she sees with applications. That episode is a good place to start with your reflection and your evaluation of your own application. You can find it at premedyears.com/288.

Because I can't actually talk to you and hear your answers, you'll need to be very honest with yourself when answering all of these questions, so you understand where you need to go from here. Also, since I go into further detail in other chapters in this book, I won't be diving deep into how to fix any potential problems in this chapter. This chapter is just a guide to get you thinking about where things may have fallen short.

It's hard to objectively evaluate your own application. You have spent a lot of time going through this process and filling out the application. Your view of your own application is too subjective. You need someone else who knows the application and the medical school admissions process to review it. They need to look over everything, give you honest criticism, and not sugarcoat it for you. As my Mappd co-founder, Rachel Grubbs, says, "Find someone who respects you more than loves you."

I have a YouTube series titled Application Renovation (applicationrenovation. com), which may help you critique your own application. In each episode of the series, I talk to a student who didn't get into medical school and review their application to look for reasons why they weren't successful. Since most students make the same mistakes, you will likely find some areas of improvement for your own application. You can apply to be on Application Renovation at applicationrenovation.com/apply.

Reviewing the Application

Let's go through the application, section by section, and think about areas where you may have fallen short. The easiest place to start is the MCAT and GPA.

MCAT

If your MCAT score is significantly below the average for matriculating medical students, that may be a very straightforward reason why you didn't get any interviews. As we've mentioned earlier in the book, the average MCAT score for matriculating MD students through AMCAS is 511.5, for TMDSAS, it's almost the same at 510.8[11], and for AACOMAS, it is a 504. If you had a 500 and only applied to MD schools, that may be a reason why you didn't get any interviews.

It's very easy for medical schools to not get to your application if they are filtering by the highest score to the lowest score. By the time they get to your application, even the schools that say they review all applications might not have any more spots available for interviewing more students.

As we talked about in the MCAT chapter, if you have a good overall MCAT score, but a very unbalanced MCAT score, meaning you scored a 123 or lower in one of the sections, that may potentially be a reason for not getting an interview as well. You may want to reach out to schools and ask if they would have filtered out your application because of that. I generally don't see many specific issues of unbalanced scores hurting applicants, but it's a question you can ask.

GPA

Just like the MCAT, if your GPA is significantly below the average for matriculating students, that is something you need to consider and potentially look at when you are re-evaluating your options. It may take another year or two,

---

11   https://www.txhex.com/_resources/docs/stats/ey19/MedStats-EY19.pdf

or more, to bring up your GPA to a competitive enough level to get an interview, and hopefully an acceptance.

The average GPA for matriculating medical students to AMCAS was 3.73, with the average science GPA being 3.66. For TMDSAS, the average GPA for matriculants was 3.80, with a science GPA of 3.73. For AACOMAS, the average GPA for undergrad students was 3.54. If your GPA is significantly lower than those averages, you may have an issue getting an interview.

Remember that your GPA story is different from everyone else's GPA story, even if they are exactly the same GPA. Your 3.5 is different than anyone else's 3.5 because of the individual trends in your grades over the course of your academic history. If you started off college with poor academic performance but finished strong, that looks better than starting strong and finishing poorly.

You can get a free two-week trial of Mappd (mappd.com) to enter all of your grades and see the trends. Mappd can also give you personalized feedback based on what you enter.

Activities

In an interview with Christine Crispin, former Dean of Admissions at UC Irvine, in Session 171 of *The Premed Years* (premedyears.com/171), her stance, and that of many other Admissions Committees, is that a lack of clinical experience is a very easy way to weed out students because they don't have enough experience to appropriately know if becoming a physician is truly right for them.

I mentioned in a previous chapter that I spoke to a student with a 3.9 GPA and 519 MCAT who didn't receive any interviews. They had zero clinical experience and no shadowing either. Their personal statement leaned on why they thought they were going to be a great physician and showed no reflection on their journey as to why they wanted to be a physician.

Another student who I talked to right around the same time was asking why they didn't get in. Their most significant "clinical" experience was working as a janitor at the hospital. They assumed that because the experience was in the hospital, it was clinical experience. Unfortunately, that's not how it works.

As you are looking through your application, evaluate if you have enough experience. It is not just a total number of hours—medical schools are oftentimes looking for consistency with those hours as well. If you gathered all of your hours early on in the application process, or early in your college career, but you don't have any hours in the last three years, that is going to be a bigger issue than someone who may have fewer total hours but has consistently been getting clinical experience over the course of that time.

If you are in the range of having at least 40 to 50 hours of shadowing and at least 100 hours of clinical experience, you'll likely have enough clinical experience, again, as long as it is consistent over a period of time.

As you are looking through your activities, did you write about them appropriately? Did you focus on your impact and talk about yourself, or did you just give basic job descriptions? Not allowing the medical school to see who you are through your activity descriptions is another potential reason why an Admissions Committee wasn't engaged enough to invite you for an interview. If so, as a reapplicant, you will need to rework your activity descriptions as much as possible while still being true to your journey and your story.

Personal Statement

Take a look at your personal statement and evaluate it. Have someone else do the same. Make sure they will be very honest with you and not try to protect your feelings. This will allow them to give you the blunt feedback you may have been missing the first time.

Does your essay answer the question, "Why do you want to be a doctor?" or is it a giant sales pitch about how you think you are going to be an amazing doctor? The personal statement needs to convey to the Admissions Committee why you want to be a doctor without selling it to them.

If you're still struggling with the personal statement even after reading the chapter in this book, and you still have not read *The Premed Playbook: Guide to the Medical School Personal Statement*, read that for a full, in-depth discussion on how to properly write a personal statement as well as over 30 personal statements with my feedback.

As a reapplicant, you should rewrite your personal statement. If you followed all of my advice in this book and in the personal statement book, and you understand your seed, you'll understand why your seed won't change, but the stories and reflections around that seed could probably be improved.

Application Timing

Sometimes your application looks great on paper, but because you applied later in the application cycle, the schools that you applied to didn't have any more space to invite you for an interview.

This is one of the biggest self-induced injuries that students make every year when it comes to applying to medical school. Students wait too long, trying to perfect every part of their application, and they don't realize the damage they are doing by delaying their application.

The later you apply, the longer the line is to be verified. This aspect of the application is most important for AMCAS. Historically, AMCAS has the longest verification times. AACOMAS, even when applying later, has historically verified applications very quickly, even in a matter of days. TMDSAS sends the applications to schools immediately and verifies afterward, so there isn't the same verification delay you would see with AMCAS or AACOMAS. With AMCAS, if you wait just a few weeks, it can change your verification time from as little as one or two weeks to four or more weeks.

If you applied late the first time, don't let it happen again. I once heard an NIH professor lecturing to premed students who said that the application process is an open book test. You know what you need to do. A late application is your first failed test of medical school. Don't fail your first open-book test.

Remember that all three of the application services open at the beginning of May. TMDSAS and AACOMAS can be submitted immediately. AMCAS has historically had a waiting period of four weeks with a submission date right around June 1st. You should be shooting for submitting your application within those first few weeks.

If you need to delay to wait for grades, to make sure you have everything set, or for something else, understand that I'm not telling you to rush a weaker application. Just like you should take the MCAT when you're ready, hit submit on your application when you think it's the best it can be. That said, don't lower your chances of acceptance by trying to make your application absolutely perfect.

I once heard a quote that a painting is never finished, it just stops in interesting places. Your application will also never be finished or perfect. You'll have to pick an interesting spot where you're comfortable stopping.

Secondary Essays

How soon were you able to turn around secondary essays? Did you let them pile up in your inbox while you went on vacation or got married? Were you so burned out by your primary application that you decided to take a break that turned into a two-month hiatus? Schools have the ability to see how long it took you to turn in your secondary essays. If you delay too long, they may assume they are last on your list and won't bother inviting you for an interview.

If you turned them in quickly, did you spend enough time on them? Did you properly research the school and provide a good enough reason why you were interested in going there? Did you provide a well-thought-out reason why they should accept you or what diversity you would bring to the class? All of those are real reasons why a medical school would pass on inviting you for an interview.

School List

When you created your school list, did you give any thought to the mission of each school and what you want out of your career? Did you only look at MCAT and GPA scores and skip over other factors like state residency, mission, and fit? Did you only apply to TMDSAS schools as an out-of-state applicant because their tuition is cheaper? Did you only apply to six MD schools with a 3.0 GPA and a 500 MCAT score?

Your school list is more important than most students realize. Many students will use the MSAR and only look at stats. Some students will use school list generator websites (Hint: Don't do this!) and apply to those schools. You have to look at each school and ask yourself *why* you want to apply there. If you don't ask yourself this before you apply, you will certainly be asked this question during your secondary application or interview, if you get that far. Do the research first and save your money if it is not a good fit.

Not applying broadly enough, especially with lower stats, and not applying to DO schools as well as MD schools, can hurt your chances of getting into medical school, too.

I Was Interviewed But Received No Acceptances

If you received an interview, that means the medical school liked your application. They liked you *enough* to invite you for an interview. They trusted your stats *enough* to assume that you would be a qualified candidate for their medical school and that you would do well in their coursework.

Some schools will only look at your interview day when determining who they are going to accept, while others may look at the complete application. It's impossible to know what happened with your specific interview and admissions decision. This is another question you might be able to ask the schools where you interviewed.

There are two scenarios. Your interview didn't hold you back, or it did. If your interview didn't hold you back, it may be the school fit, stats, or something else that left you a little short of the goal line. If it did hold you back, it could mean you are not a good interviewer, or you just had a bad day. Just like a bad personal statement can derail your application, a bad interview can easily get you a rejection. I interviewed Natalie on *The Premed Years* after she was finally accepted to medical school during her third application cycle. During her second cycle, she had six interviews, and she was waitlisted at all of them. This screams interview issues to me.

Luckily, interviewing is a skill that can be improved. Natalie signed up for a set of mock interviews with me. Her first one was rough. She was doing everything wrong. Over the course of the next few mock interviews, however, she started to focus on the right things, and for her third application cycle, she had six acceptances instead of six waitlists. You can listen to that interview at premedyears.com/241. Ultimately, she went from trying to prove she was going to be great, to just being herself and having a great conversation.

Don't forget to get a copy of my book, *The Premed Playbook: Guide to the Medical School Interview,* to help you focus on the right things.

WHEN TO REAPPLY

One of the biggest mistakes students make is reapplying to medical school too soon. Once it is late enough in the application cycle for you to realize you're not going to get in, there are usually only a couple of months until the new application cycle opens.

If you didn't get into medical school, you need to take the time to reflect on that, and then get feedback on your applications from schools, advisors, and mentors. They should provide criticism on the areas where you need to improve your application for the next time.

Jumping right back into the application cycle doesn't give you enough time to improve your application. Just like rushing a MCAT retake, it shows medical schools that you are not taking the time to reflect and improve. If you have a lot of areas to improve, it will be hard to know when you will be ready. You can check out Mappd's series, "Am I Ready?", created to specifically answer this question at amiready.tv.

Sometimes jumping right back in may be appropriate. If you believe, after looking at the different sections of your application, that everything looked good but maybe you just applied late, or your MCAT score wasn't very good but you retook it and it's much improved, then potentially reapplying will be okay. If those two data points suggest the reason why you didn't get in, and those two things are now fixed, reapplying might be a good choice.

Most of the time, though, it's going to be a lack of clinical experience, poor GPA or poor trending GPA, or other things that are going to take time to fix in your application. Taking another year to work on those things is usually the right answer. One thing to remember is that your MCAT score is usually only good for three years, and if you need to take the time to fix your application, that may mean taking the MCAT again.

Being on this side of medical school and the application process, I can tell you that one more year is not a big deal. That said, before medical school and your medical career, one year can seem like an eternity. When you sit back and think about delaying your application a year or reapplying again with the same mistakes and not getting in again, it makes much more sense to just take the time to fix your application appropriately and then push forward the following application cycle, or whenever you are ready again.

It's Not Over

Remember that needing to reapply after not getting any interviews does not mean you can't be a doctor.

Being rejected or waitlisted at every school where you interviewed does not mean you won't be an amazing physician either.

Reapplying to medical school only means you didn't put together the right story with the right stats this time. Make sure you don't do it again, and you'll set yourself up for success in the future.

Being a reapplicant is also not a scarlet letter that will hurt your chances in the future. There is a lot of misinterpretation of the available data stating that reapplicants have a much lower chance of being accepted. People misinterpret the data and state that being a reapplicant causes the lower acceptance rates. This isn't necessarily true. Reapplicants already had something wrong with their application in the first place. Many students don't put in the work and reflection needed to improve their application before applying again, resulting in another cycle of rejections.

If you have to reapply, don't let that "reapplicant status" get you down.

GAP YEARS

While not specifically application related, I want to talk about gap years because you may be planning them or may need to take them if your application cycle doesn't go as planned. If you read the previous chapter and you decide that yes, I'm going to delay my application, then you need to start asking yourself, "What do I want to do during my gap year?"

Let's start with, what is a gap year? Taking a gap year means that you are not directly starting medical school within a year of graduating college. For example, if you graduate college in the Winter of 2029 and you don't start medical school (meaning you didn't apply in the Summer of 2029) in 2030, then you are taking a gap year. Remember that you need to apply to medical school the year before you plan to start. This is a confusing part of the application process for many, which leads to unintended gap years.

A gap year can help you work on your MCAT score, improve your GPA trend, give you time to get more experience, or just give you a break from being a student. There are no right or wrong reasons to want to take a gap year. There may be wrong ways to spend a gap year, though.

If you are taking a gap year to travel the world and go backpacking in Europe without adding anything to your clinical experiences, this could hurt your application. While backpacking and seeing the world would be an amazing experience, if you are completely stepping away from your premed path to do it, this may look like a red flag to Admissions Committees. You may be 100% convinced that this is what you want to do, and you've racked up a ton of hours doing everything you can to reassure yourself that you want to be a physician, but if you have a year where you are doing nothing medically related, some doubt may form in the minds of the Admissions Committee members. Are you just having fun, or are you a little burned out? Are you starting to question things? Are you going to make it through medical school?

That's not to say that your gap year needs to be 100% filled with clinical experience, volunteering, and shadowing. I was talking with a student recently about their gap year opportunities and wondering if they should go back into the hospital where they were certified as an anesthesia tech, or if they should do something fun like work at the zoo. I said, "Why can't you do both?" You don't have to work full-time in a hospital providing full-time patient care. If you are not hurting for hours, and if you have a lot of clinical experience already, you don't need to spend the year padding your résumé. You need to spend a year enjoying yourself, but also keep a foot in the world of medicine, showing consistency and proving to yourself and to the medical schools where you are applying that this is what you want.

I love the phrase, "Actions speak louder than words." I get a lot of pushback from students who see me talk about this on social media. They think that if they are certain they want to be a physician, they should be allowed to do whatever they want during a gap year, including traveling the world and not getting any more clinical experience. Their words, on the application, will say they want to be a physician, but their actions will say something else. That is what I want you to avoid.

Do Gap Years Hurt my Chances of Getting into Medical School?

Contrary to your parents' belief that if you take a gap year, your life and career are over, taking a gap year can actually benefit you tremendously in several different ways. The first is that it will likely benefit you psychologically. Taking a break from school, clearing your head, getting away from the books, and allowing yourself to breathe and rejuvenate is always a good thing. Your gap year can also help you address some of the shortcomings in your application.

Your parents' biggest fear is that you are going to take a gap year and fall out of love with medicine and in love with being a hobo traveling around the country in a VW bug, but that is not something that you need to worry about. If that happens, that is okay, and that is just your path. You and your parents shouldn't assume that just because you are taking a gap year, you are going to run away from medicine altogether.

Medical schools don't necessarily care whether or not you take a gap year. More and more students are coming in at an older age, either after taking gap years or switching careers after being in the workforce. Gap years are becoming more and more common amongst premeds applying to medical school.

Gap Years Don't Help Your Application

I need to clear up one very common myth right now. Students are seeing that more students getting into medical school have taken a gap year, so they assume that taking a gap year is helping the applicants and that medical schools want to see that. Remember, correlation does not equal causation. We cannot broadly say that gap years help applicants. What we can say is there are many reasons why someone would take a gap year, and what they do during that gap year could strengthen the weaknesses in their application.

It is not the gap year that matters—it is what they have done in their entire premed journey, including their gap year. You may have a solid application without needing to take a gap year. Don't take one just because you think it will help your application. Take one if you think you have weaknesses in your application that need further development or if you need a break before applying.

YOU'VE GOT THIS

The medical school application cycle brings with it a mix of emotions. I want to congratulate you for taking the first step and getting this book to help get you going in the right direction. Too many students, including myself the first time I applied, think that applying to medical school is just as easy as applying to college. Fill out some paperwork, submit your application, and let the acceptances start rolling in. Unfortunately, it's not that easy.

You know that now. You are prepared to put together a great application. You now know you need to show the Admissions Committees who you are and not just what you've done.

Sometimes, even with a great application, medical schools may tell you no. What you need to remember is that they are not telling you that you can't be a medical student or a great physician. They are simply telling you that you can't do it this year.

For most of you, you'll get that magical acceptance to medical school. Congratulations and welcome to the family!

Rejection or acceptance, I'm proud of each and every one of you for putting in the time and effort to enter this amazing profession. We need you. You are our future.

ABOUT THE AUTHOR

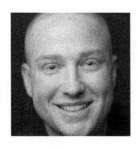

Dr. Ryan Gray is a former United States Air Force Flight Surgeon who found a passion for helping premed students on their journey to medical school. Best known for his podcasts, which have been downloaded over 10,000,000 times, Dr. Gray has interviewed numerous Admissions Committee members and deans of admissions for medical schools.

Through *The Premed Years* podcast and the Medical School Headquarters sites, Dr. Gray has helped hundreds of thousands of students gain the confidence they require to successfully navigate the premed path.

Dr. Gray co-founded Mappd, the only tool of its kind to help you navigate your premed journey at mappd.com. Use it to track all of your courses, activities, MCAT prep, letter writers, and more. You can even invite your premed advisor to view your data to provide better feedback during your meetings.

Dr. Gray lives outside of Boulder, CO, with his wife Allison, who is a Neurologist, and their children Hannah, and Ethan. Dr. Gray is also a Clinical Instructor at the University of Colorado School of Medicine.

If you'd like Dr. Gray to speak to your premed club or at your conference, send an email to team@medicalschoolhq.net.

RESOURCES

For a full list of resources, including links to specific episodes and videos about different topics I covered in this book, go to medschoolapplicationbook.com/resources.

Websites

medicalschoolhq.net—Medical School Headquarters: For the best information to help premeds on the path to medical school.

mappd.com—Mappd: Track and navigate your premed journey.

premedhangout.com—Join an amazing group of collaborative premed students.

Podcasts

premedpodcasts.com—There are many podcasts on the Meded Media Network: The Premed Years, OldPreMeds Podcast, The MCAT Podcast, Specialty Stories, The MCAT CARS Podcast, Ask Dr. Gray: Premed Q&A, Inside Health Education, Ask the Dean, The Short Coat Podcast, and more coming!

YouTube

premed.tv—If you'd prefer YouTube videos over podcasts, Dr. Gray has you covered there as well. Check out his growing library of videos!

mappd.tv—More great videos and discussion with the Mappd team.

One-on-One Advising

If you're looking for more personalized help on your journey to medical school, I've put together an amazing advising team at mappd.com/services. We can help with your primary application, secondary applications, interview prep, and general premed questions.

CPSIA information can be obtained
at www.ICGtesting.com
Printed in the USA
JSHW041503240421
13915JS00018B/18